Demystifying Polyneuropathy - Recent Advances and New Directions

Edited by Patricia Bozzetto Ambrosi

Published in London, United Kingdom

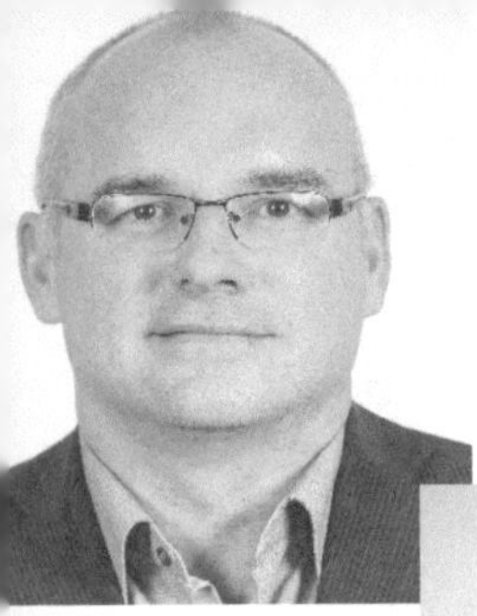
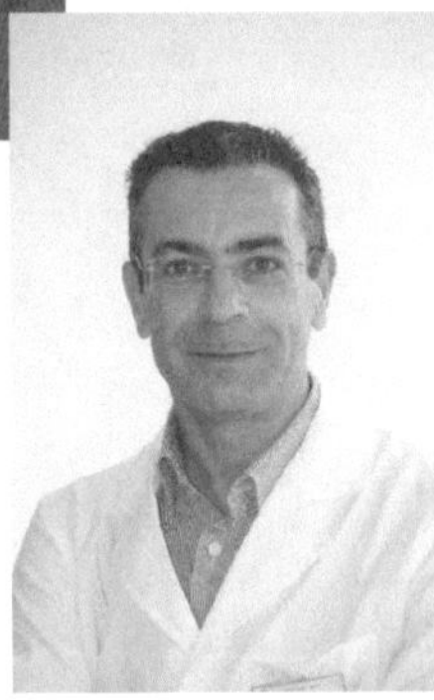
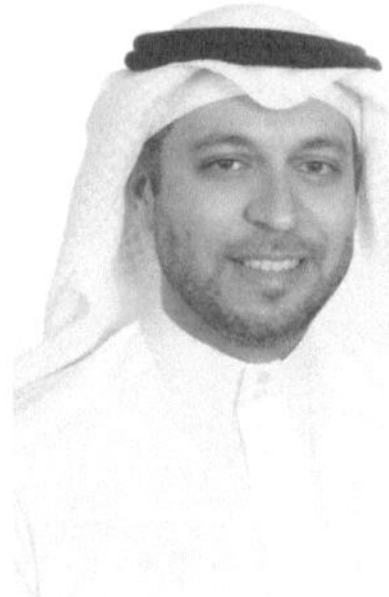
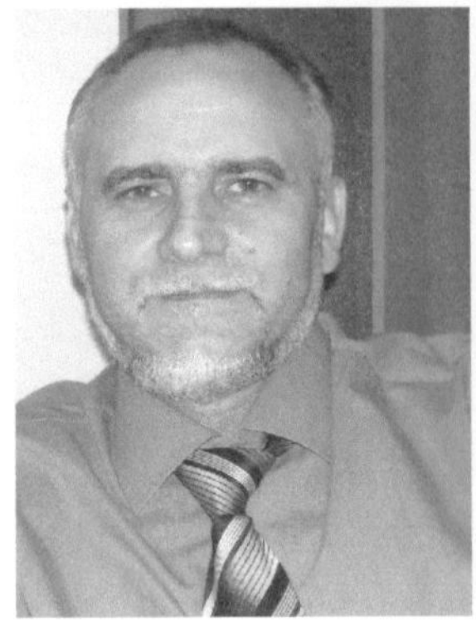
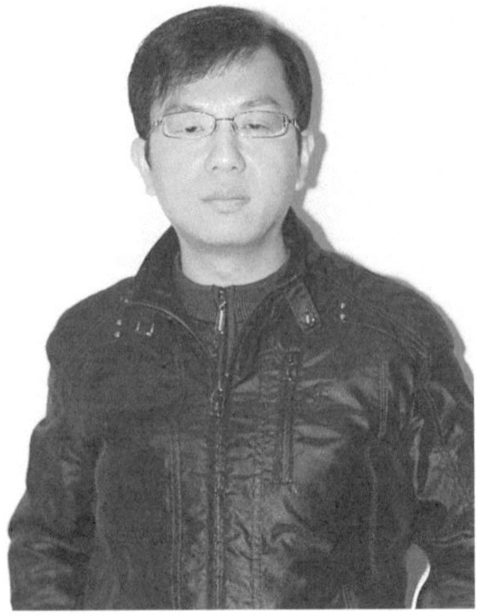
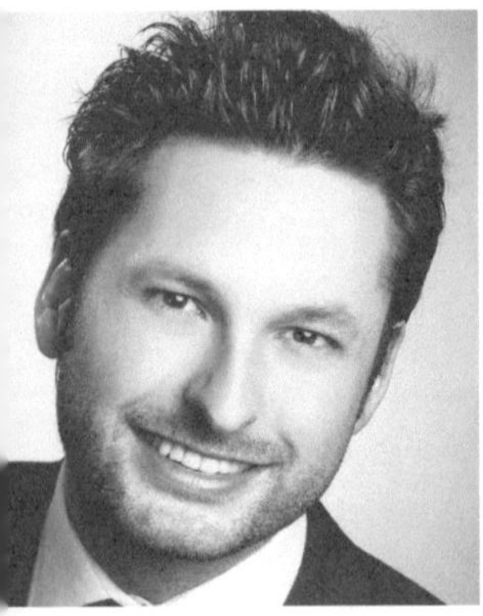
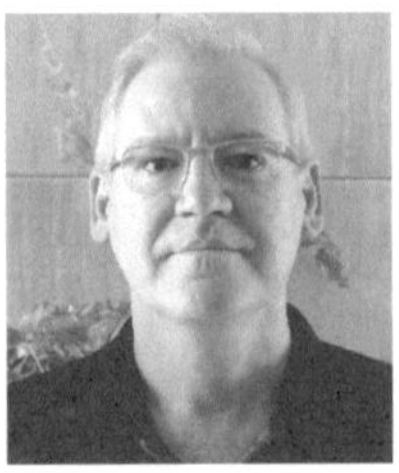

IntechOpen

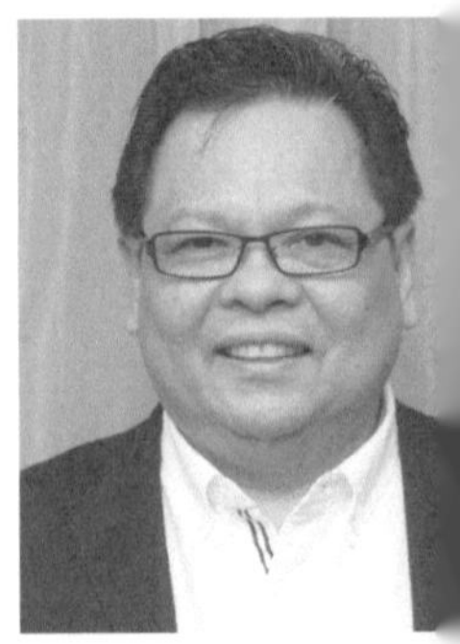
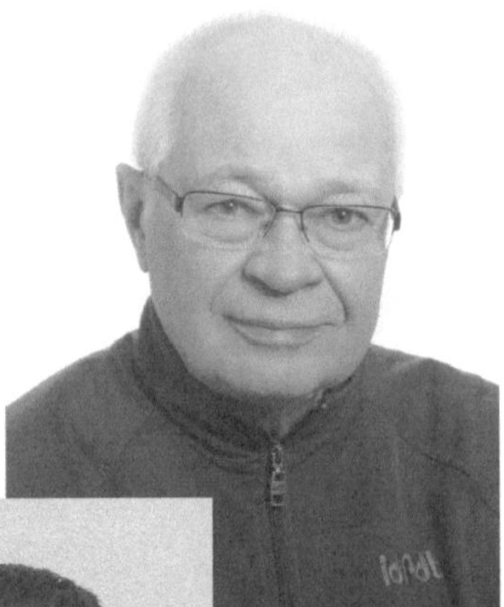
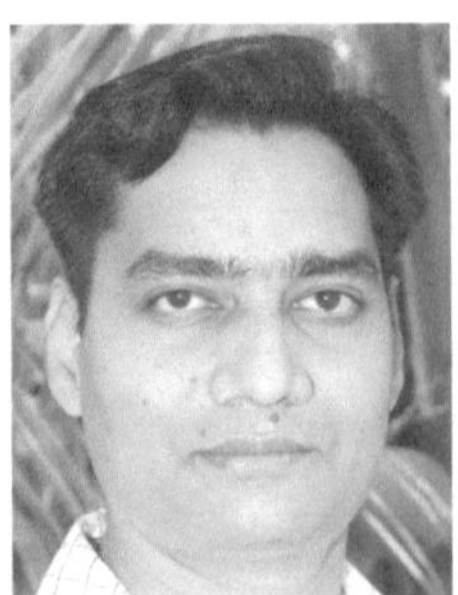
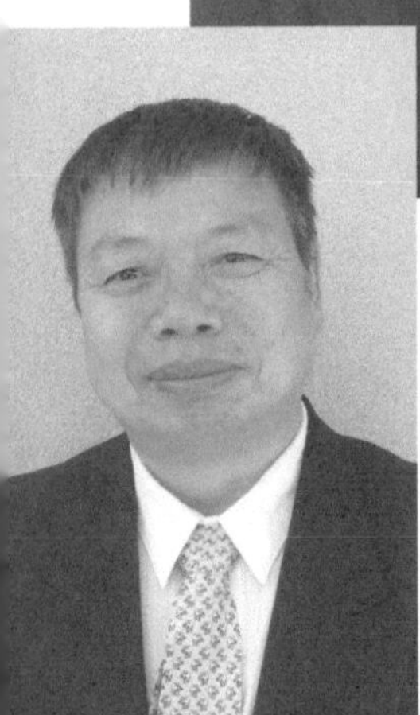
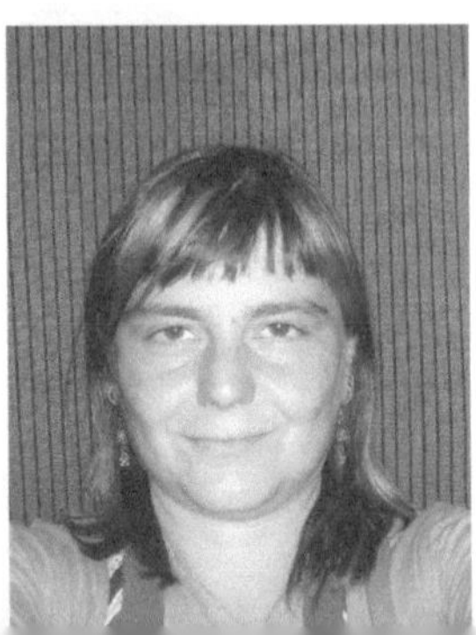
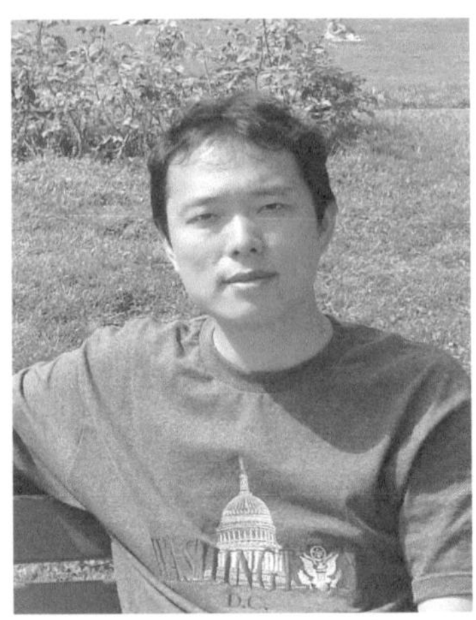

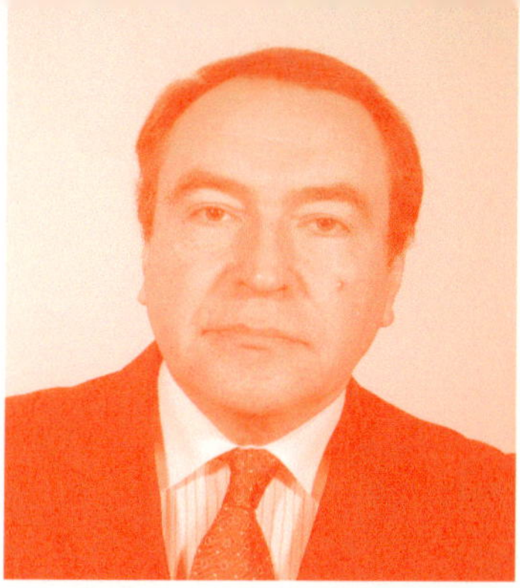
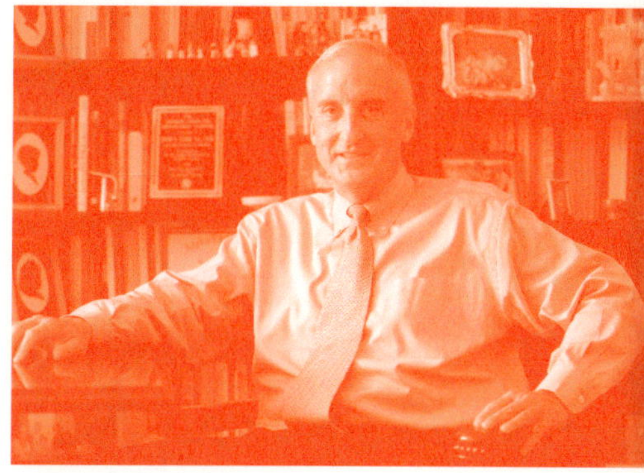
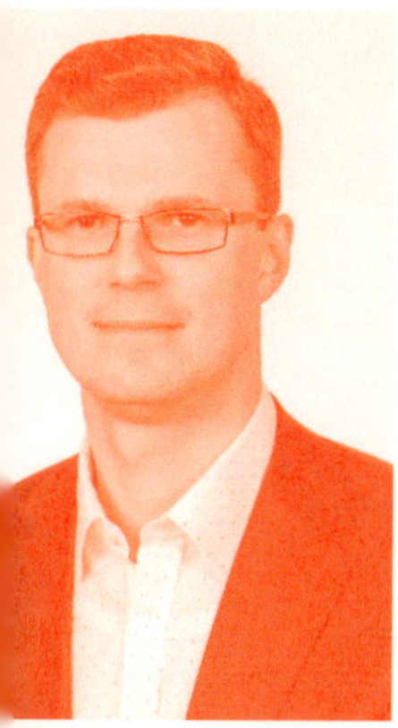
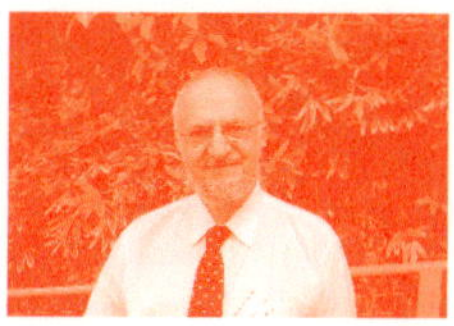
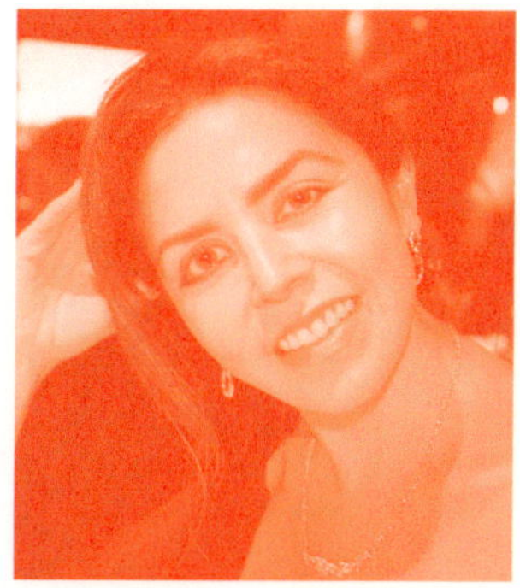

Supporting open minds since 2005

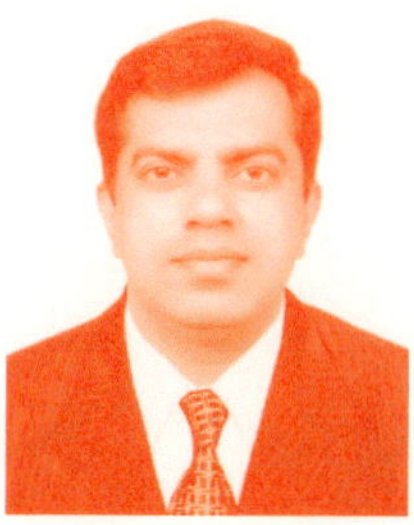
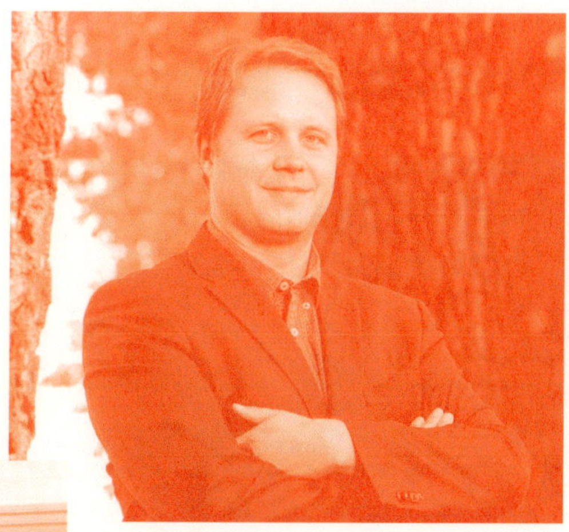
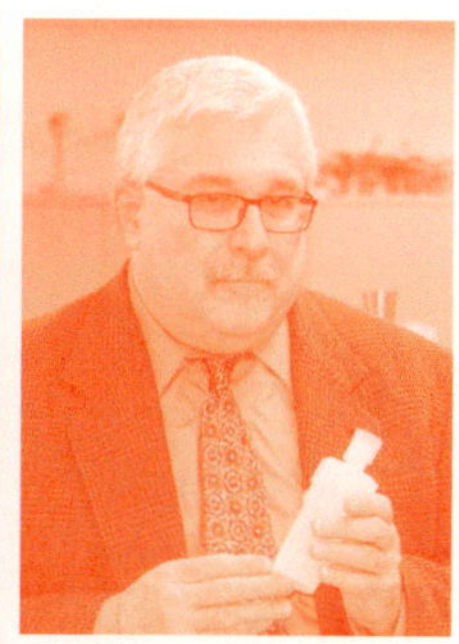
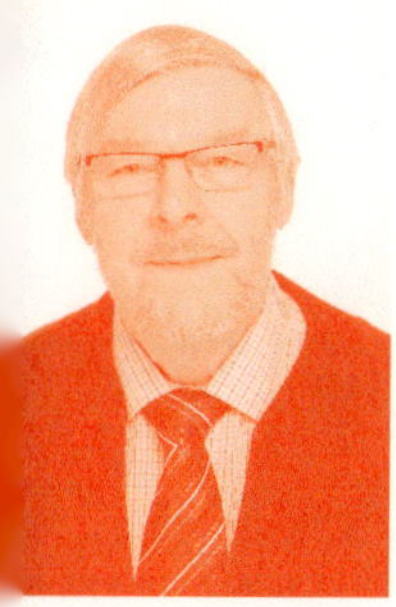
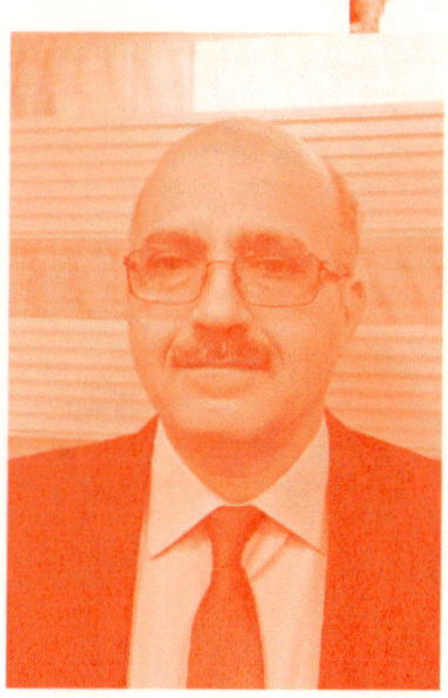
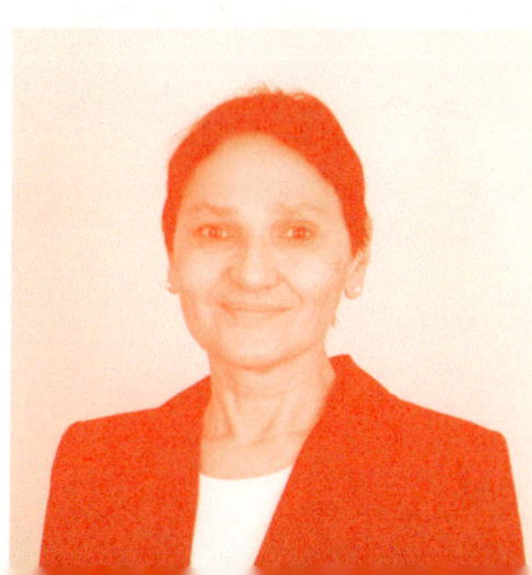
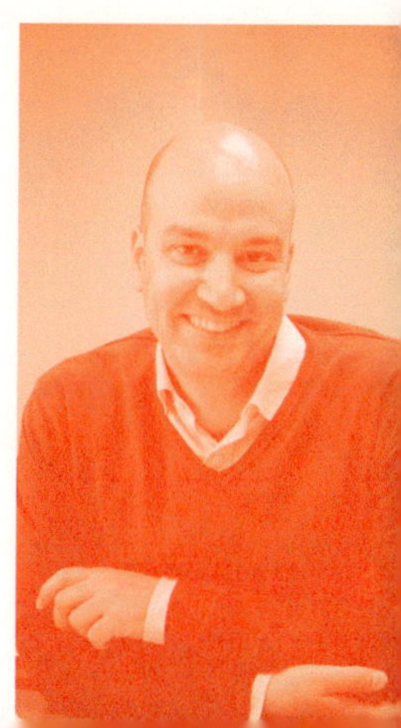

Demystifying Polyneuropathy - Recent Advances and New Directions
http://dx.doi.org/10.5772/intechopen.73946
Edited by Patricia Bozzetto Ambrosi

Contributors
Mikel Sánchez, Diego Delgado, Ane Garate, Pello Sánchez, Nicolás Fiz, Jorge Guadilla, Juan Azofra, Beatriz Aizpurua, Ane Miren Bilbao, Jaime Oraa, Fernando Yangüela, Gokhan Ozdemir, José Antonio A. Vega, Yolanda Garcia-Mesa, Jorge Garcia-Piqueras, Giussepina Salvo, Juan L. Cobo, Olivia García-Suarez, Elda Alba, Jorge Feito, Mouna Snoussi, Faten Frikha, Zouhir Bahloul, Fitri Octaviana, Ahmad Yanuar Safri, Darma Imran, Patricia Price

First published in London, United Kingdom, 2019 by IntechOpen
IntechOpen is the global imprint of INTECHOPEN LIMITED, registered in England and Wales, registration number: 11086078, The Shard, 25th floor, 32 London Bridge Street
London, SE19SG - United Kingdom
Printed in Croatia

British Library Cataloguing-in-Publication Data
A catalogue record for this book is available from the British Library

Additional hard and PDF copies can be obtained from orders@intechopen.com

Demystifying Polyneuropathy - Recent Advances and New Directions
Edited by Patricia Bozzetto Ambrosi
p. cm.
Print ISBN 978-1-83881-191-4
Online ISBN 978-1-83881-192-1
eBook (PDF) ISBN 978-1-83881-193-8

Meet the editor

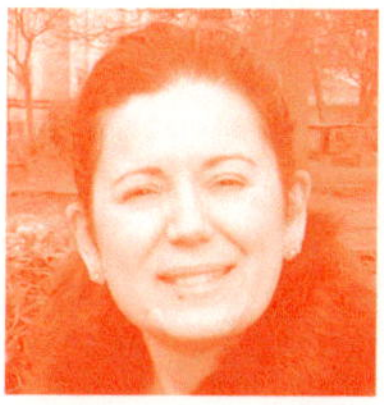

Dr. Bozzetto Ambrosi completed her neurology and neurosurgery training at the Hospital da Restauracao, Recife, Brazil, in 2008 followed by specialization in medical imaging and diagnostic and therapeutic neuroradiology at Pierre and Marie Curie University in Paris, France, respectively, in 2011 and 2014. She was previously a visiting professor at Beaujon University Hospital in Paris, France. Dr. Ambrosi is dedicated, driven, and passionate about providing the highest standard of service for patients. She has extensive experience of working in a wide range of prestigious neurological and neuroscience centers all over the world with more than 20 years of rich experience in medical assistance, research, and development, as well as teaching and mentoring in the field of neurology. She has excellent communication and writing skills, with a keen interest in new technologies, research, and publication in neurosciences. She is proficient in several languages and has experience in peer reviewing and editorship in the medical field covering various topics in national and international journals. Her expertise is in identifying the best strategy, integrating teamwork, and executing work with a strong determination based on knowledge. She has excellent presentation and interpersonal skills with proven abilities in teaching and training for various academic and professional appointments. Presently, she is an independent consultant and professor in neurology/neuroradiology and neurosurgery.

Contents

Preface

Polyneuropathy is a distinct term for a generalized and relatively homogenous process that affects many peripheral nerves, but it is the distal nerves that are generally more affected by the disorder at large. It also commonly encompasses any disturbance of the peripheral nervous system, including radiculopathies and mononeuropathies and/or disorders involving the nerves of the central and peripheral nervous system. In daily practice, the wide variety of causes must be identified in obtaining a diagnosis and polyneuropathies should be differentiated from other diseases of the peripheral nervous system, including mononeuropathies and multiplex mononeuropathy (multifocal neuropathy) and some disorders of the central nervous system. Central nervous system diseases such as brain tumor, stroke, or spinal cord injury occasionally present symptoms that are difficult to distinguish from polyneuropathies.

The complex structure and function of nerves of the nervous system make them susceptible to a variety of inflammatory, hereditary, infectious, toxicity, and other factors that can impair their health and function, leading to the clinical disorder of polyneuropathy. Although there is a lack of population-based studies, researchers generally agree that no specific cause is identified in up to half of cases of patients with polyneuropathy at referral centers despite deeper investigations.

There are no simple rules one can apply to reliably distinguish the type of polyneuropathy produced by various disease categories (e.g., demyelinating versus axonal, chronic versus acute, and sensory versus motor). The interest in more reliable instruments to apply to diseases involving nerves of the nervous system has become a significant part of the full investigation to clarify the etiologic diagnosis of polyneuropathy. Regarding its management, although several procedures involving conservative and surgical interventions are available, promising biological strategies are needed to open new horizons so the drawbacks of these challenging conditions may be overcome.

Knowledge about polyneuropathy has advanced on all fronts, significantly, through education and inspirational leadership. Contributors to this first edition of *Demystifying Polyneuropathy - Recent Advances and New Directions* are many of these leaders, and their writing and creativity are remarkable. The authors are practitioners and researchers with an inestimable amount of experience, and they share their knowledge and wisdom, seeking not only to teach but also to inspire those who will follow them. They point out not only what we already know but also what we need to discover, thereby directing a path toward observation, service, and experimentation, each of which is integral to the study of polyneuropathy in imminent and future directions.

As editor, and on behalf of the authors and assistants, I extend my gratitude to the publisher for striking visual content to help create a comprehensive book, complete with unique topic selections, so that the blend of academic and other content is at once logical and stimulating. At this point, I am enormously grateful to the extraordinary team at IntechOpen, including Edi Lipović, Mirena Calmić, and

Maja Božičević. My publishing editorship family always sets the bar high, patiently helping me by leaps and bounds to achieve a finished book. And, definitely, my academic family has embraced this exciting experience while my own little family graciously has allowed me the time to pursue this lovely undertaking.

Finally, I am excited to introduce you, the reader, to our endeavor, shared in three main sections, five chapters in total. In the first section, general considerations and diagnostic approach are discussed through the chapter, The Cutaneous Biopsy for the Diagnosis for the Peripheral Neuropathies: Meissner's Corpuscles and Merkel's, which highlight skin biopsy as an alternative method of peripheral nerve biopsy for the analysis of nerve involvement in the differential of polyneuropathy. Given the relative simplicity of the technique and its ability to provide quantitative data, the test is also likely to be useful in following disease progression or response to treatment. The chapter provides us a comprehensive rationale concerning this method within neuropathies and an update of the available information in this topic.

In the second section, Etiologies and Pathogenesis, three chapters are included: the first is on HIV-associated neuropathy: the clinical picture of what is triggered by HIV infection and other maladies is very similar; it includes neuropathic pain, tingling sensation, and numbness. Several related aspects are discussed. The second chapter explains how peripheral neuropathy in connective tissue diseases is characterized by different organ disorders due to the loss of immune system tolerance to autoantigens. Peripheral neuropathy is one of the features of these diseases with variable, and it is often seen in the course of the disease. The chapter reviews the clinical, diagnostic, and therapeutic features associated with the common diffuse connective tissue diseases, and it presents future directions. A third innovative chapter is presented about a new definition of a nonclassified polyneuropathy condition called 'working hand syndrome.'

In the third section, Management and New Clinical Applications, a final chapter discusses platelet-rich plasma for injured peripheral nerves. Although polyneuropathy is among the most challenging categories of neurological diseases, effective forms of treatment for polyneuropathy have been introduced over the last decades. Biological therapies are promising using conservative and surgical approaches. Effects mechanisms, clinical guidelines, protocols, and results from bench to bedside are fully described.

We wish to thank those who contributed to these new insights into polyneuropathy. Particularly, we acknowledge our contributing authors for their excellent submissions to this book, and our patients, families, friends, and collaborators for their help and patience at each step in the production of this book. In summary, we hope you enjoy this wonderful reading, and we are proud to have you join us in this unique and new experience.

Patricia Bozzetto Ambrosi
Paris Diderot University,
France

Section 1

General Considerations and Diagnostic Approach

Chapter 1

The Cutaneous Biopsy for the Diagnosis of Peripheral Neuropathies: Meissner's Corpuscles and Merkel's Cells

Olivia García-Suárez, Yolanda García-Mesa, Jorge García-Piqueras, Giuseppina Salvo, Juan L. Cobo, Elda Alba, Ramón Cobo, Jorge Feito and José A. Vega

Abstract

Cutaneous biopsy is a complementary method, alternative to peripheral nerve biopsy, for the analysis of nerve involvement in peripheral neuropathies, systemic diseases, and several pathologies of the central nervous system. Most of these neuropathological studies were focused on the intraepithelial nerve fibers (thin-myelinated Aδ fibers and unmyelinated C fibers), and few studies investigated the variations in dermal innervation, that is, large myelinated fibers, Merkel's cell-neurite complexes, and Meissner's corpuscles. Here, we updated and summarized the current data about the quantitative and qualitative changes that undergo MCs and MkCs in peripheral neuropathies. Moreover, we provide a comprehensive rationale to include MCs in the study of cutaneous biopsies when analyzing the peripheral neuropathies and aim to provide a protocol to study them.

Keywords: skin biopsy, peripheral neuropathy, Meissner's corpuscles, Merkel's cells

1. Introduction

Since the last half of the past century, the analysis in the cutaneous biopsy of nerves, Merkel's cells (MkCs), and sensory corpuscles, especially Meissner's corpuscles (MCs), become a complementary method to diagnose peripheral neuropathies [1] and a reliable alternative to peripheral nerve biopsy. Nevertheless, it has been during the last decade that numerous studies have provided consistent evidence to support this technique as a valuable tool to understand the etiologies of some neurological diseases and to follow up clinical trials [2–4] (**Figures 1** and **2**).

Most of the neuropathological studies on cutaneous biopsies were focused on intraepithelial nerve fibers, which are thin-myelinated Aδ fibers or unmyelinated C fibers [2, 3, 5–9]. Conversely, few studies have investigated the large myelinated fibers (although it can offer notable advantages over the unmyelinated ones [10]). Also, the quantitative and qualitatively changes in MCs and MkCs associated to peripheral neuropathies are poorly known although the study of MCs has gained interest [11–13].

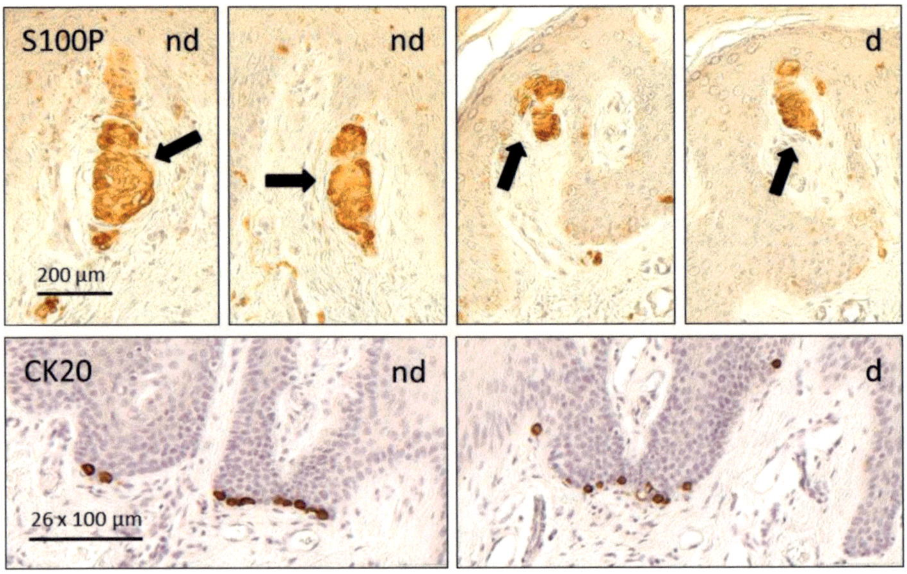

Figure 1.
Meissner's corpuscles (arrows) and Merkel's cells in the first toe skin of nondiabetic (nd) and diabetic (d) subjects as observed using immunohistochemistry for S100 protein (S100P) and cytokeratin-20 (CK20), specific markers for lamellar cells and Merkel's cells, respectively.

The evaluation of the dermal innervation, including large fibers, MCs, and MkCs, is not currently included within the routine analysis of skin biopsies because of the lack of a validated protocol. Changes in the density and size of MC and MkCs (i.e., variations in number/unit of surface, atrophy and/or hypertrophy, protein expression, etc.), can reflect quantitative or qualitative variations in the number of sensory neurons or nerve fibers innervating them or in the cells forming MCs themselves. Even more, they might also reflect pathologies of the central nervous system, and in these cases, the cutaneous biopsy becomes a method to study diseases difficult to be analyzed without invasive surgery.

This chapter is aimed to update the current data about the quantitative and qualitative changes in MCs and MkCs in peripheral neuropathies, as well as to provide a comprehensive rationale to include them in the study of cutaneous biopsies when analyzing the peripheral neuropathies. Furthermore, our purpose is to provide a technical protocol for analyzing MCs and MkCs in cutaneous biopsies. We have excluded from this review the intraepidermic nerve fibers because they have been extensively studied in peripheral neuropathies, and standardized method has been proposed and accepted [4, 9].

2. State of the art: a review and update of the literature

2.1 Why do we study Meissner's corpuscles and Merkel's cells for clinical purposes

The cutaneous MCs are sensory structures placed just beneath the epidermis within the dermal papillae in areas especially sensitive to light touch, like the fingertips, palms, soles, lips, and male and female genital skin [14–16]. They show an ellipsoid morphology with the main axis perpendicular to the skin surface and a size largely variable (length of 80–150 µm and diameter of 20–40 µm). Structurally, they consist of an axon that runs between the stacked nonmyelinating Schwann-like cells (the so-called lamellar cells) and habitually lacks a differentiated capsule [14, 16, 17].

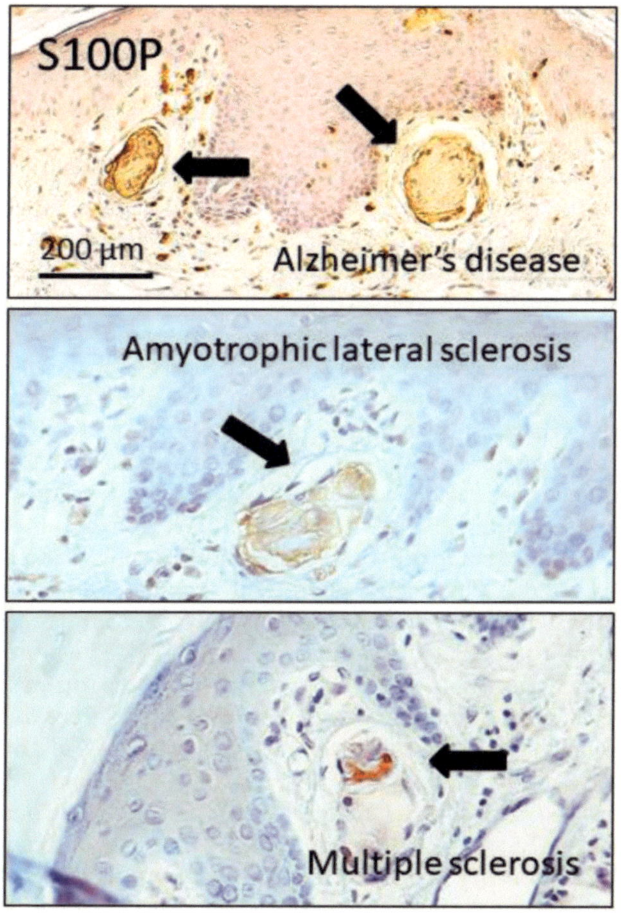

Figure 2.
Meissner's corpuscles (arrows) of the palmar aspect of the fingers of patients diagnosed of Alzheimer's disease, amyotrophic lateral sclerosis, and multiple sclerosis, as observed using immunohistochemistry for S100 protein (S100P). The samples were obtained during necropsy and in compliance with Spanish law.

MCs are particularly abundant in the fingers and palm hand, which are two zones easily accessible for biopsy. Nevertheless, the analysis of MCs from these zones has many problems. First of all, the normal density (MCs/mm^2) at this localization should be determined to compare normal and pathological conditions. The most ancient studies established that the density of MCs in the human hand is ~10–24 MCs/mm^2 [18–20], it is higher in the fingertip (2.7/mm^2 $\pm$ 0.68) than in the palm (1.33/mm^2 $\pm$ 0.6), and it does not change significantly with age [21]. Nolano et al. [22] found 33.02/mm^2 $\pm$ 13.2 in the fingertip of digit III and 45/mm^2 in the digit V; Herrmann et al. [12] determined that the density of MCs on the palmar side of digit V is 12/mm^2 $\pm$ 5.3, whereas in the skin of the thenar eminence, it is 5.1/mm^2 $\pm$ 2.2.

The second trouble for the use of MCs in the diagnosis of neuropathies is whether or not MCs change in density and characteristic with aging. A reduction in number and size of MCs in elderly is generally assumed [18, 23–25], but detailed studies are not available. Preliminary data from our laboratory demonstrate that aging is accomplished of a reduction in the number and size of digital MCs, as well as changes in their architecture and immunohistochemical properties (García-Piqueras et al., unpublished). However, the variations in the corpuscular size and morphology of MCs are difficult to evaluate because of their large variability within the same skin sample. Therefore, in the absence of evident atrophy, hypertrophy, or corpuscular disruption, the evaluation of these parameters must be cautiously considered when evaluating cutaneous biopsies.

The main constituents of MCs, that is, the axon and lamellar cells, contain specific proteins as widely demonstrated using immunohistochemistry [17, 26, 27]. These studies reported a large volume of information, but they are purely descriptive and do not consent to quantify those proteins and their possible variations in neuropathies. The central axon displays immunoreactivity for general neuronal markers (neuron-specific enolase, protein gene product 9.5, neurofilament subunit proteins). They also express Ca^{2+}-binding proteins such as calbindin D28k, parvalbumin, calretinin, and neurocalcin, which presumably regulate the axonic Ca^{2+} homeostasis and therefore participate in the mechanoelectric transduction. Recently, our research's group detected axonic TRPC6, TRPV4, ASIC2, and Piezo2 ion channels that work as putative mechanoproteins [28–30]. Regarding lamellar cells, the vimentin is the intermediate filament filling their cytoplasm, while the glial fibrillary acidic protein is always absent. They strongly express S100 protein colocated with parvalbumin or calbindin D-28 kDa. The lamellar cells also display immunoreactivity for TrkB, the signaling receptor for the neurotrophins BDNF/NT-4 [31]. Apart from axon- or lamellar cell-specific proteins, there are some others shared by both corpuscular constituents. They include p75NTR and TrkA (low-affinity pan-neurotrophin receptor and the high-affinity receptor for nerve growth factor, respectively; [32, 33]), the epidermal growth factor receptor [34], or cell death protein Bcl-2 [35]. The presence of some ion channels in the lamellar cells has been also reported [28–30]. It is possible that some of these proteins undergo changes during peripheral neuropathies, but limited information is so far available in this topic (see [17]). The proteins present in human MCs are summarized in **Table 1**.

The cutaneous MkCs are special epidermal cells placed in the basal layer of the epidermis, isolated or forming clusters, in both the glabrous and hairy skin. They are innervated by Aβ sensory axons connected through synapse-like contacts forming the so-called MkCs-neurite complexes. MkCs are involved in fine touch working as a part of slowly adapting type I low-threshold mechanoreceptors and express specific mechanoproteins [16, 30, 36–39]. MkCs have an epithelial origin and do not originate from the neural crest, as classically accepted [40–42].

Using immunohistochemistry, diverse proteins have been detected in the MkC-neurite complexes. They include low-molecular-weight cytokeratins and a repertory of synaptic vesicles-related proteins (chromogranin A, synaptophysin), different neuropeptides as well as neurotransmitter receptors, neurotrophin receptors, ion channels (ASIC2 and Piezo2), and neuron-specific enolase [28, 43–46]. The axon of the MkC-neurite complexes displays immunoreactivity for general neuronal markers (**Table 1**).

The density of MCs varies from an anatomical region to another, and it is directly related to the sensibility of those zones [47]. In terms of density as far as we know, no age-dependent changes have been communicated. Recently, we have found significant reduction in of digital MkCs with aging (García-Piqueras et al., unpublished). On the other hand, whether or not MkCs, or the nerve fibers innervating them, are involved in peripheral neuropathies has been poorly studied, but this possibility should be explored because the easily accessibility to MkCs-neurite complexes.

2.2 Variations in MCs and MKCs in peripheral neuropathies

Data reporting changes in MCs in peripheral neuropathies are scarce and are restricted to diabetes and other rare inheretary neuropathies, HIV infection, mechanical or traumatic nerve entrapment, and a miscellaneous group of systemic diseases with neurological symptoms.

	Meissner's corpuscles		**Merkel's cell-neurite complex**	
Protein	**Ax**	**LC**	**Ax**	**MC**
Axonal proteins				
Neuron-specific enolase	■		■	■
Protein gene product 9.5	■		■	
β-Arrestin 1	■			
GAP-43	■			
Ca2+-binding proteins				
S100 protein		■		
Calbindin D28K	■	■		
Calretinin	■	■		
Neurocalcin	■			
Cytoskeletal proteins				
Neurofilament proteins	■		■	
Vimentin		■		
Growth factor receptors				
p75NTR (pan-neurotrophin receptor)	■	■		■
TrkA (NGF receptor)	■	■		■
TrkB (BDNF/NT4 receptor)		■		
EGF receptor		■		
Putative mechanoproteins (ion channels)				
ASIC2	■		■	■
Piezo2	■			■
TRPC6	■			
TRPV4	■	■		■
TRPM8				■
Cell death-live proteins				
Bcl-2	■	■		
Neuropeptides and bioactive amines				
Serotonin				■
Bombesin				■
Vasoactive intestinal polypeptide				■
Substance P				■
CCK8				■
Calcitonin gene-related peptide				■
Neuropeptide receptors				
NMDA				■
Synaptic vesicle-associated proteins				
Chromogranin A				■
Synaptophysin				■

Table 1.
Proteins detected in human Meissner's corpuscles and Merkel's cell neurite complexes using immunohistochemistry. Red: positivity for a protein in the axon of Meissner's corpuscles; Blue: positivty for a protein in the lamellar cells (LC) of Meissner's corpuscles.

2.2.1 Diabetic neuropathy

Distal symmetric peripheral neuropathy is one of the most common complications of diabetes [48] and involves motor, autonomic, and sensory nerve fibers. The histopathological studies have provided evidence that both the thin unmyelinated C fibers and the large myelinated ones are affected in on diabetic neuropathy. Consistently, the two most prominent complaints are peripheral pain and changes in touch [13, 49–52]. The intraepidermic nerve fibers as well as the nerve apparatus of the dermis are reduced in the diabetic neuropathy, and the reduction of the dermic nerves involves MCs. Importantly, although some authors have argued their interest in studying MCs and MkCs to better understand the diabetic neuropathy [53], only few studies have approached this topic.

In cutaneous biopsies, it was shown that the density of MCs is significantly reduced in diabetic patients with respect to the controls (10.2 ± 8.4 vs. $16.2 \pm 9.4/\text{mm}^2$, more evidently in type I than in type II diabetes), and this correlated with a reduction in median and ulnar nerves sensory amplitude; moreover, some MCs were hypertrophic or showed anomalies in their architecture (disorganization of the lamellar cells and increase in the irregularity of the axons) [54]. Similar findings as those obtained from cutaneous biopsy were observed using *in vivo* reflectance confocal microscopy at the thenar eminence and digit V [55]. We have recently communicated that long-term diabetic neuropathy courses with a reduction in the number and size of MCs and changes in their immunohistochemical profile [56] (**Figure 1**).

Nevertheless, the number and size of MCs are probably related with the time of evolution of the neuropathy. In fact, in an animal model of diabetes that develop neuropathy, MCs were found more abundant and hypertrophic during the first few years of hyperglycemia, whereas after a long time, the hypertrophy declines but the number of corpuscles remained higher than in age-matched nondiabetic subjects; furthermore, the MCs from the diabetic animals found had abnormal structure and immunochemistry properties [57].

On the other hand, as far as we know, the only study reporting a reduction in the number of immunohistochemically demonstrable MkCs in diabetic neuropathy was from our laboratory [56].

2.2.2 Charcot-Marie-Tooth disease

Charcot-Marie-Tooth (CMT) disease is a common inherited neuromuscular disorder characterized by neuropathies without known metabolic alterations. In the skin of patients with common and rare forms of CMT caused by different mutations, the density of MCs is reduced compared with normal controls [58–60]. Similar findings were reported by Almodovar et al. [61] using *in vivo* reflectance confocal microscopy.

2.2.3 Human immunodeficiency virus (HIV) neuropathy

HIV-sensory neuropathy is a common complication of HIV infection and may be associated with significant morbidity due to neuropathic pain [62]. Several approaches exist for quantitative assessment of human HIV-associated distal sensory polyneuropathy, and some of them have analyzed both unmyelinated and myelinated nerve fibers, as well as MCs. Using *in vivo* reflectance confocal microscopy, it was found a marked reduction in MCs [12, 63] in HIV+ subjects with and without distal sensory neuropathy [64].

2.2.4 Entrapment neuropathies

Surprisingly, little is known about the impact of entrapment neuropathy on target innervation. More than 20 years ago, we reported that human digital MCs survive to entrapment or section of peripheral nerves for more than 10 years, and although its number remains relatively stable, denervated MCs lack some antigens or change the pattern of expression of some others [65–67]. These data were confirmed recently in subjects undergoing carpal tunnel syndrome [68].

2.2.5 Miscellaneous

A reduction in density or loss of MCs has also been reported in the skin of patients suffering from Ross syndrome (a rare disorder of sweating associated with areflexia and tonic pupil) [69], POEMS syndrome (polyneuropathy, organomegaly, endocrinopathy, monoclonal gammopathy, and skin changes) [70], systemic sclerosis [71], pachyonychia congenita (in contrast, MkC densities are higher) [72], chronic inflammatory demyelinating polyradiculoneuropathy [73], and systemic lupus erythematosus [12].

2.3 MCs are also altered in central nervous system disorders

In addition to the abovementioned peripheral neuropathies, changes in MCs have been reported in Parkinson's disease associated or not with dementia [74–76], spinobulbar muscular atrophy [77], Friedreich's ataxia [78], amyotrophic lateral sclerosis [79], or Guillain-Barré syndrome [73]. Furthermore, altered cutaneous innervation also has been observed in some psychiatric disorders [80] and mental deficiencies [81] (**Figure 2**).

3. Proposal of a method to systematically study MCs and MkCs in cutaneous biopsies

MCs are only present in glabrous skin, and therefore fingers or toes are appropriate regions to take cutaneous biopsies focused to evaluate them; in spite of the discrepancies regarding their density in these places, they are abundant enough.

In our opinion, the palmar aspect of fingertip IV would be an ideal region to be biopsied, because it is not involved in handling; the lateral borders should be excluded to avoid damaging the digital nerves and the formation of neuromas. On the other hand, toe pad biopsies can be also useful, but they contain a lower density of MCs than fingers [82].

The Joint Task Force EFNS/PNS [9] recommends to perform a 3 mm punch skin biopsy (including epidermis and the subpapillary and reticular dermis), using a sterile technique and under local anesthesia. A sample of these dimensions does not need sutures, heal completely within 1 week, and this normally guaranties no side effects or complaints. Informed consent is required, and information on the possible risks must be always provided. The fixation of the skin samples is recommended in 2% PLP (2% paraformaldehyde, 0.075 M lysine, 0.037 M sodium phosphate, 0.01 M periodate) or Zamboni's solution. We have also obtained excellent structural results and good antigen preservation using Bouin's fixative and buffered 10% formaldehyde. Conversely, 4% paraformaldehyde masked most of the antigens present in MCs. The thickness of the sections is also important. The Joint Task Force EFNS/

PNS especially recommends 50-μm thick sections to perform 3D reconstructions of MCs. Nevertheless, our experience demonstrates that to demonstrate the occurrence of most antigens present in the axon or in the lamellar cells of Meissner's corpuscles, 8 or 10 μm sections are appropriate.

There are different techniques for identification and assessment of MCs (silver impregnation techniques, electron microscopy, immunohistochemistry, and immunofluorescence), but the ideal one should allow to the quantification and specific immunostaining, distinguishing the different MCs constituents. In routine studies, at least one marker for the axon and one for the lamellar cells should be used. Indirect immunofluorescence, especially when associated with confocal microscopy, provides an opportunity to investigate multiple neuronal and nonneuronal proteins within the same MC and also to perform its 3D reconstruction using appropriate computerized image analysis systems. Ideally, double immunostaining for both axon and lamellar cells, associated or not with labeling of the nuclei, provides a global image of the morphology and size of the corpuscle, as well as of the arrangement of corpuscular constituents (**Figure 3**).

To quantify MCs, we use the method proposed by Verendeev et al. [83] to establish the density of MCs in the fingertips of primates. Briefly, 10-μm-thick sections, 200 μm apart, processed for S100 protein immunohistochemistry, are used. The sections are scanned by SCN400F scanner (Leica, Leica Biosystems™) and computerized using SlidePath Gateway LAN software (Leica, Leica Biosystems™). Then, in each section, MCs are identified and counted by two independent observers. The average numerical values were corrected applying the Abercrombie's formula: $N = n^*T/(T + H)$, where N is the corrected average number of MCs, n is the counted average number of MCs in all sections of a fingertip, T is the average section's thickness, and H is the average diameter of the counted MCs. Through a specific tool of the abovementioned software, the average MCs diameter was determinate measuring the horizontal axis by drawing a straight line approximately in the central region of each corpuscle. The longitudinal epidermis of each section (mm) is measured with the same tool, and the average length was multiplied by the section's thickness (mm) to give the measured surface area (mm^2). Finally, the average number of Meissner corpuscles (N) was divided by the surface area (mm^2) that is the density of MCs by squared millimeter of skin (number of MCs/mm^2) (**Figure 4**). To establish the density of digital Merkel's cells, we used the same method immunostaining Merkel's cells for cytokeratin.

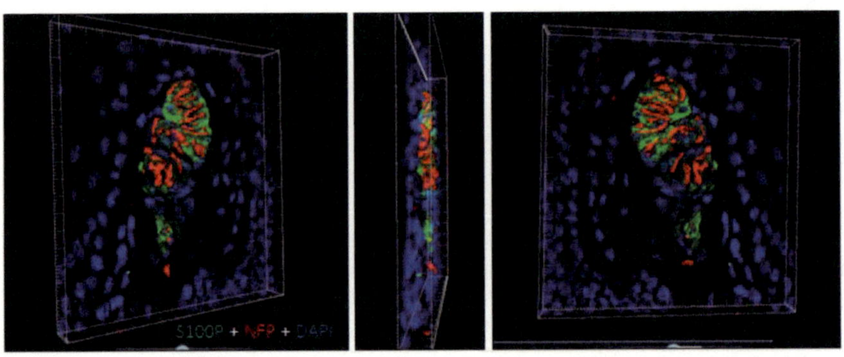

Figure 3.
3D reconstruction of a Meissner's corpuscle in a finger of a 25-year-old male. The axon is labeled in red, and the lamellar cells in green. The cell nuclei were labeled with DAPI. Scale bar = 20 μm.

DOI: http://dx.doi.org/10.5772/intechopen.81687

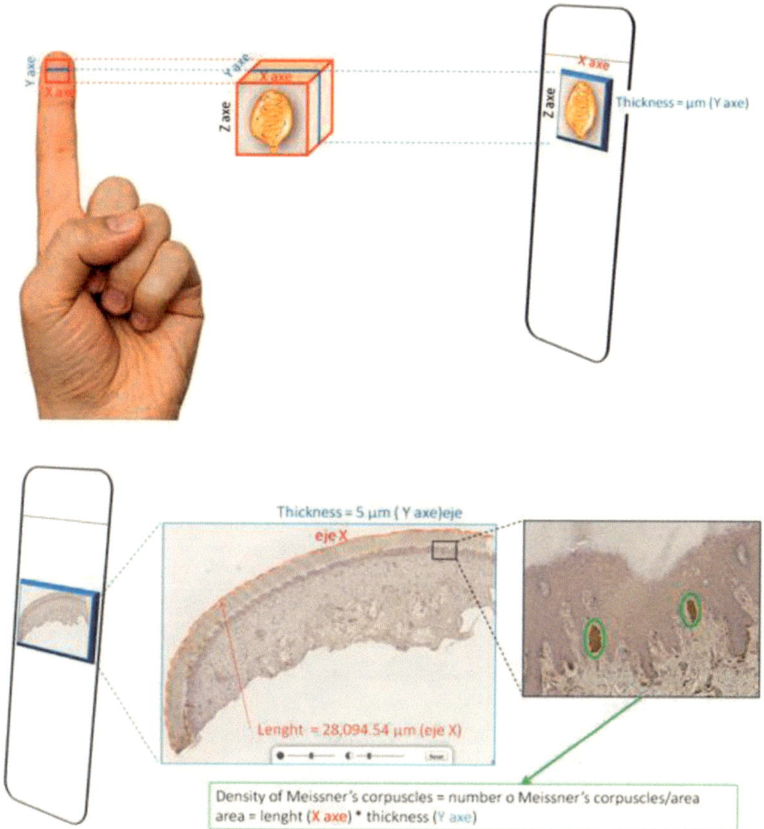

Figure 4.
Schematic representation of the technical procedure to quantify Meissner's corpuscles in sections of human digital skin immunostained for the detection of S100 protein.

4. Final remarks and future prospectives

Peripheral neuropathies are diverse and require a multidimensional approach for detection and monitoring clinical and research setting. The minimal invasiveness of skin biopsy makes it a useful tool not only for diagnostics but also for following the progression or the effects of a treatment in neuropathies.

Pathophysiological studies in patients with large nerve fiber polyneuropathies are limited because the difficulty in obtaining nerve samples due to the invasive nature of the procedure. For this reason, some authors utilized skin biopsies to obtain morphological and molecular information from large dermal myelinated nerve fibers. The development of new methods to evaluate skin innervation, including MCs, through noninvasive techniques, that is, in vivo reflectance confocal microscopy, may contribute to better understand the changes in sensory corpuscles in neuropathies [12, 55, 61, 84–86].

Nevertheless, to use MCs as a complementary method in the diagnosis of neurological diseases, more studies are still necessary. Firstly, the density of MCs must be mapped in the specific areas where they are abundant and easily accessible to cutaneous biopsy, especially the hand glabrous skin. Secondly, the physiological age-related changes in the number and protein composition of MCs of these selected areas must be established. Quantitative data, apart from qualitative, on changes in protein composition of MCs with aging are necessary as a baseline for possible pathological changes. In addition to immunohistochemical studies, skin biopsy is amenable to the extraction of mRNA, RT-PCR, or microarrays for genes involved in neuropathies, and these methods should be used and standardized to study MCs. Finally, future studies should include not only neuropathies such as neurofibromatosis [85], or other rare metabolic neuropathies such as Gaucher type 1 disease [86], but also central nervous system diseases such as Alzheimer's disease.

Author details

Olivia García-Suárez[1], Yolanda García-Mesa[1], Jorge García-Piqueras[1], Giuseppina Salvo[1], Juan L. Cobo[1,2], Elda Alba[3], Ramón Cobo[1], Jorge Feito[1,4] and José A. Vega[1,5]*

1 Departamento de Morfología y Biología Celular, Grupo SINPOS, Universidad de Oviedo, Spain

2 Servicio de Cirugía Máxilofacial, Hospital Universitario Cental de Astrias, Oviedo, Spain

3 Servicio de Neurología, Hopital Universitario "La Paz", Madrid, Spain

4 Servicio de Anatomía Patológica, Complejo Hospitalario de Salamanca, Salamanca, Spain

5 Facultad de Ciencias de la Salud, Universidad Autónoma de Chile, Santiago de Chile, Chile

*Address all correspondence to: javega@uniovi.es

References

[1] Dyck PJ, Winkelmann RK, Bolton CF. Quantitation of Meissner's corpuscles in hereditary neurologic disorders. Charcot-Marie-Tooth disease, Roussy-Levy syndrome, Dejerine-Sottas disease, hereditary sensory neuropathy, spinocerebellar degenerations, and hereditary spastic paraplegia. Neurology. 1966;**16**:10-17

[2] Sommer C. Skin biopsy as a diagnostic tool. Current Opinion in Neurology. 2008;**21**:562-568

[3] Lauria G, Lombardi R. Small fiber neuropathy: Is skin biopsy the holy grail? Current Diabetes Reports. 2012; **12**:384-392

[4] Mellgren SI, Nolano M, Sommer C. The cutaneous nerve biopsy: Technical aspects, indications, and contribution. Handbook of Clinical Neurology. 2013; **115**:171-188

[5] Lauria G, Devigili G. Skin biopsy as a diagnostic tool in peripheral neruropathy. Nature Clinical Practice. Neurology. 2007;**3**:546-557

[6] Sommer C, Lauria G. Skin biopsy in the management of peripheral neuropathy. Lancet Neurology. 2007;**6**: 632-642

[7] Lauria G, Lombardi R, Camozzi F, Devigili G. Skin biopsy for the diagnosis of peripheral neuropathy. Histopathology. 2009;**54**:273-385

[8] Lauria G, Bakkers M, Schmitz C, Lombardi R, Penza P, Devigili G, et al. Intraepidermal nerve fiber density at the distal leg: A worldwide normative reference study. Journal of the Peripheral Nervous System. 2010;**15**: 202-207

[9] Lauria G, Hsieh ST, Johansson O, Kennedy WR, Leger JM, Mellgren SI, et al. European Federation of Neurological Societies/Peripheral Nerve Society Guideline on the use of skin biopsy in the diagnosis of small fiber neuropathy. Report of a joint task force of the European Federation of Neurological Societies and the Peripheral Nerve Society. European Journal of Neurology. 2010;**17**:903-912, e44-9

[10] Saporta MA, de Moraes Maciel R. Analysis of myelinating Schwann cells in human skin biopsies. Methods in Molecular Biology. 2018;**1739**:359-369

[11] Dyck PJ. Enumerating Meissner corpuscles: Futute gold standard of large fiber sensoriomotor polyneuropathy? Neurology. 2007;**69**:2116-2118

[12] Herrmann DN, Boger JN, Jansen C, Alessi-Fox C. In vivo confocal microscopy of Meissner corpuscles as a measure of sensory neuropathy. Neurology. 2007;**69**:2121-2127

[13] Myers MI, Peltier AC, Li J. Evaluating dermal myelinated nerve fibers in skin biopsy. Muscle & Nerve. 2013;**47**:1-11

[14] Munger BL, Ide C. The structure and function of cutaneous sensory receptors. Archives of Histology and Cytology. 1988;**51**:1-34

[15] Zelena J. Nerves and Mechanoreceptors. London: Chapman & Hall; 1994

[16] Zimmerman A, Bai L, Ginty DD. The gentle touch receptors of mammalian skin. Science. 2014;**346**: 950-954

[17] Vega JA, López-Muñiz A, Calavia MG, García-Suárez O, Cobo J, Otero J, et al. Clinical implication of Meissner's corpuscles. CNS & Neurological Disorders Drug Targets. 2012;**11**: 856-868

[18] Bolton CF, Winkelmann RK, Dyck PJ. A quantitative study of Meissner's corpuscles in man. Neurology. 1966;**16**: 1-9

[19] Halata Z, Munger BL. The terminal myelin segments of afferent axons to cutaneous mechanoreceptors. Brain Research. 1985;**347**:177-182

[20] Johnson KO, Yoshioka T, Vega-Bermudez F. Tactile functions of mechanoreceptive afferents innervating the hand. Journal of Clinical Neurophysiology. 2000;**17**:539-558

[21] Kelly EJ, Terenghi G, Hazari A, Wiberg M. Nerve fiber and sensory end organ density in the epidermis and papillary dermis of human hand. British Journal of Plastic Surgery. 2005;**58**: 774-779

[22] Nolano M, Provitera V, Crisci C. Quantification of myelinated endings and mechanoreceptors in human digital skin. Annals of Neurology. 2003;**54**: 197-205

[23] Ridley A. Silver staining of nerve endings in human digital glabrous skin. Journal of Anatomy. 1969;**104**:41-48

[24] Bruce MF. The relation of tactile thresholds to histology in the fingers of elderly people. Journal of Neurology, Neurosurgery, and Psychiatry. 1980;**43**: 730-734

[25] Iwasaki T, Goto N, Goto J, Ezure H, Moriyama H. The aging of human Meissner's corpuscles as evidenced by parallel sectioning. Okajimas Folia Anatomica Japonica. 2003;**79**:185-189

[26] Vega JA, Haro JJ, Del Valle ME. Immunohistochemistry of human cutaneous Meissner and Pacinian corpuscles. Microscopy Research and Technique. 1996;**34**:351-361

[27] Vega JA, García-Suárez O, Montaño JA, Pardo B, Cobo JM. The Meissner and Pacinian sensory corpuscles revisited new data from the last decade. Microscopy Research and Technique. 2009;**72**:299-309

[28] Cabo R, Alonso P, Viña E, Vázquez G, Gago A, Feito J, et al. ASIC2 is present in human mechanosensory neurons of the dorsal root ganglia and in mechanoreceptors of the glabrous skin. Histochemistry and Cell Biology. 2015; **143**:267-276

[29] Alonso-González P, Cabo R, San José I, Gago A, Suazo IC, García-Suárez O, et al. Human digital Meissner corpuscles display immunoreactivity for the multifunctional ion channels Trpc6 and Trpv4. Anatomical Record (Hoboken). 2017;**300**:1022-1031

[30] García-Mesa Y, García-Piqueras J, García B, Feito J, Cabo R, Cobo J, et al. Merkel cells and Meissner's corpuscles in human digital skin display Piezo2 immunoreactivity. Journal of Anatomy. 2017;**231**:978-989

[31] Calavia MG, Feito J, López-Iglesias L, de Carlos F, García-Suarez O, Pérez-Piñera P, et al. The lamellar cells in human Meissner corpuscles express TrkB. Neuroscience Letters. 2010;**468**: 106-109

[32] Vega JA, Del Valle ME, Haro JJ, Calzada B, Suarez-Garnacho S, Malinovsky L. Nerve growth factor receptor immunoreactivity in Meissner and Pacinian corpuscles of the human digital skin. The Anatomical Record. 1993;**236**:730-736

[33] Vega JA, Vazquez E, Naves FJ, Del Valle ME, Calzada B, Represa JJ. Immunohistochemical localization of the high-affinity NGF receptor (gp140-trkA) in the adult human dorsal root and sympathetic ganglia and in the nerves and sensory corpuscles supplying digital skin. The Anatomical Record. 1994;**240**:579-588

[34] Vega JA, Vazquez E, Naves FJ, Calzada B, del Valle ME, Represa JJ. Expression of epidermal growth factor receptor (EGFr) immunoreactivity in human cutaneous nerves and sensory corpuscles. The Anatomical Record. 1994;**240**:125-130

[35] González-Martínez T, Monjil DF, Aguado-Barrios A, Cobo J, Germanà G, Vega JA. Bcl-2 immunoreactivity in human cutaneous Meissner and Pacinian corpuscles. Neuroscience Letters. 2006;**394**:13-16

[36] Woo SH, Lumpkin EA, Patapoutian A. Merkel cells and neurons keep in touch. Trends in Cell Biology. 2015;**25**: 74-81

[37] Feng J, Luo J, Yang P, Du J, Kim BS, Hu H. Piezo2 channel-Merkel cell signaling modulates the conversion of touch to itch. Science. 2018;**360**: 530-533

[38] Maricich SM, Wellnitz SA, Nelson AM, Lesniak DR, Gerling GJ, Lumpkin EA, et al. Merkel cells are essential for light-touch responses. Science. 2009; **324**:1580-1582

[39] Maksimovic S, Nakatani M, Baba Y, Nelson AM, Marshall KL, Wellnitz SA, et al. Epidermal Merkel cells are mechanosensory cells that tune mammalian touch receptors. Nature. 2014;**509**:617-621

[40] Morrison KM, Miesegaes GR, Lumpkin EA, Maricich SM. Mammalian Merkel cells are descended from the epidermal lineage. Developmental Biology. 2009;**336**:76-83

[41] Van Keymeulen A, Mascre G, Youseff KK, Harel I, Michaux C, De Geest N, et al. Epidermal progenitors give rise to Merkel cells during embryonic development and adult homeostasis. The Journal of Cell Biology. 2009;**187**:91-100

[42] Woo SH, Stumpfova M, Jensen UB, Lumpkin EA, Owens DM. Identification of epidermal progenitors for the Merkel cell lineage. Development. 2010;**137**: 3965-3971

[43] Sieber-Blum M, Szeder V, Grim M. The role of NT-3 signaling in Merkel cell development. Progress in Brain Research. 2004;**146**:63-72

[44] Boulais N, Pereira U, Lebonvallet N, Gobin E, Dorange G, Rougier N, et al. Merkel cells as putative regulatory cells in skin disorders: An in vitro study. PLoS One. 2009;**4**(8):e6528

[45] Maksimovic S, Baba Y, Lumpkin EA. Neurotransmitters and synaptic components in the Merkel cell-neurite complex, a gentle-touch receptor. Annals of the New York Academy of Sciences. 2013;**1279**:13-21

[46] Isgrò MA, Bottoni P, Scatena R. Neuron-specific enolase as a biomarker: Biochemical and clinical aspects. Advances in Experimental Medicine and Biology. 2015;**867**:125-143

[47] Kim DK, Holbrook KA. The appearance, density, and distribution of Merkel cells in human embryonic and fetal skin: Their relation to sweat gland and hair follicle development. The Journal of Investigative Dermatology. 1995;**104**:411-416

[48] Vinik AI, Nevoret ML, Casellini C, Parson H. Diabetic neuropathy. Endocrinology and Metabolism Clinics of North America. 2013;**42**:747-787

[49] Bierhaus A, Haslbeck KM, Humpert PM, Liliensiek B, Dehmer T, Morcos M, et al. Loss of pain perception in diabetes is dependent on a receptor of the immunoglobulin superfamily. The Journal of Clinical Investigation. 2004; **114**:1741-1751

[50] Bril V, Buchanan RA. Long-term effects of ranirestat (AS-3201) on

peripheral nerve function in patients with diabetic sensorimotor polyneuropathy. Diabetes Care. 2006; **29**:68-72

[51] Christianson JA, Ryals JM, Johnson MS, Dobrowsky RT, Wright DE. Neurotrophic modulation of myelinated cutaneous innervation and mechanical sensory loss in diabetic mice. Neuroscience. 2007;**145**:303-313

[52] Obrosova IG, Stavniichuk R, Drel VR, Shevalye H, Vareniuk I, Nadler JL, et al. Different roles of 12/15-lipoxygenase in diabetic large and small fiber peripheral and autonomic neuropathies. The American Journal of Pathology. 2010;**177**:1436-1447

[53] Alsunousi S, Marrif HI. Diabetic neuropathy and the sensory apparatus "Meissner corpuscle and Merkel cells". Frontiers in Neuroanatomy. 2014;**8**:79

[54] Peltier AC, Myers MI, Artibee KJ, Hamilton AD, Yan Q, Guo J, et al. Evaluation of dermal myelinated nerve fibers in diabetes mellitus. Journal of the Peripheral Nervous System. 2013;**18**: 162-167

[55] Creigh PD, McDermott MP, Sowden JE, Ferguson M, Herrmann DN. In-vivo reflectance confocal microscopy of Meissner's corpuscles in diabetic distal symmetric polyneuropathy. Journal of the Neurological Sciences. 2017;**378**: 213-219

[56] García-Mesa Y, García-Piqueras J, Feito J, Cabo R, Vega JA, García-Suárez O. Evaluation of Meissner corpuscles and Merkel cells in diabetic neuropathy. European Journal of Clinical Investigation. 2018;**48**(Sup. 1):195-196

[57] Paré M, Albrecht PJ, Noto CJ, Bodkin NL, Pittenger GL, Schreyer DJ, et al. Differential hypertrophy and atrophy among all types of cutaneous innervation in the glabrous skin of the monkey hand during aging and naturally occurring typ. 2 diabetes. The Journal of Comparative Neurology. 2007;**501**:543-567

[58] Saporta MA, Katona I, Lewis RA, Masse S, Shy ME, Li J. Shortened internodal length of dermal myelinated nerve fibres in Charcot-Marie-Tooth disease typ. 1A. Brain. 2009;**132**(Pt 12): 3263-3273

[59] Manganelli F, Nolano M, Pisciotta C, Provitera V, Fabrizi GM1, Cavallaro T, et al. Charcot-Marie-Tooth disease: New insights from skin biopsy. Neurology. 2015;**85**:1202-1208

[60] Nolano M, Manganelli F, Provitera V, Pisciotta C, Stancanelli A, Caporaso G, et al. Small nerve fiber involvement in CMT1A. Neurology. 2015;**84**:407-414

[61] Almodovar JL, Ferguson M, McDermott MP, Lewis RA, Shy ME, Herrmann DN. In vivo confocal microscopy of Meissner corpuscles as a novel sensory measure in CMT1A. Journal of the Peripheral Nervous System. 2011;**16**:169-174

[62] Aziz-Donnelly A, Harrison TB. Update of HIV-associated sensory neuropathies. Current Treatment Options in Neurology. 2017;**19**:36

[63] Herrmann DN. Noninvasive and minimally invasive detection and monitoring of peripheral neuropathies. Expert Review of Neurotherapeutics. 2008;**8**:1807-1816

[64] Almodovar JL, Schifitto G, McDermott MP, Ferguson M, Herrmann DN. HIV neuropathy: An in vivo confocal microscopic study. Journal of Neurovirology. 2012;**18**: 503-510

[65] Albuerne M, López S, Naves FJ, Martínez-Almagro A, Represa J, Vega JA. S100α and S100β proteins in human cutaneous sensory corpuscles: Effects of

nerve and spinal cord injury. The Anatomical Record. 1998;**251**:351-359

[66] Márquez J, Pérez-Pérez M, Naves FJ, Vega JA. Effect of spinal cord and peripheral nerve injury on human cutaneous sensory corpuscles. An immunohistochemical study. Journal of the Peripheral Nervous System. 1997;**2**: 49-59

[67] López SM, Pérez-Pérez M, Márquez JM, Naves FJ, Represa J, Vega JA. p75 and TrkA neurotrophin receptors in human skin after spinal cord and peripheral nerve injury, with special reference to sensory corpuscles. The Anatomical Record. 1998;**251**:371-383

[68] Schmid AB, Bland JD, Bhat MA, Bennett DL. The relationship of nerve fibre pathology to sensory function in entrapment neuropathy. Brain. 2014;**137** (Pt 12):3186-3199

[69] Nolano M, Provitera V, Perretti A, Stancanelli A, Saltalamacchia AM, Donadio V, et al. Ross syndrome: A rare or a misknown disorder of thermoregulation? A skin innervation study on 12 subjects. Brain. 2006;**129**: 2119-2131

[70] Santoro L, Manganelli F, Bruno R, Nolano M, Provitera V, Barbieri F. Sural nerve and epidermal vascular abnormalities in a case of POEMS syndrome. European Journal of Neurology. 2006;**13**:99-102

[71] Provitera V, Nolano M, Pappone N, di Girolamo C, Stancanelli A, Lullo F, et al. Distal degeneration of sensory and autonomic cutaneous nerve fibres in systemic sclerosis. Annals of the Rheumatic Diseases. 2005;**64**:1524-1526

[72] Pan B, Byrnes K, Schwartz M, Hansen CD, Campbell CM, Krupiczojc M, et al. Peripheral neuropathic changes in pachyonychia congenita. Pain. 2016; **157**:2843-2853

[73] Hutton EJ, Carty L, Laura M, Houlden H, Lunn MP, Brandner S, et al. c-Jun expression in human neuropathies: A pilot study. Journal of the Peripheral Nervous System. 2011;**16**: 295-303

[74] Nolano M, Provitera V, Estraneo A, Selim MM, Caporaso G, Stancanelli A, et al. Sensory deficit in Parkinson's disease: Evidence of a cutaneous denervation. Brain. 2008;**131**:1903-1911

[75] Nolano M, Provitera V, Manganelli F, Iodice R, Stancanelli A, Caporaso G, et al. Loss of cutaneous large and small fibers in naive and l-dopa-treated PD patients. Neurology. 2017;**89**(8):776-784

[76] Ikemura M, Saito Y, Sengoku R, Sakiyama Y, Hatsuta H, Kanemaru K, et al. Lewy body pathology involves cutaneous nerves. Journal of Neuropathology and Experimental Neurology. 2008;**67**:945-953

[77] Manganelli F, Iodice V, Provitera V, Pisciotta C, Nolano M, Perretti A, et al. Small-fiber involvement in spinobulbar muscular atrophy (Kennedy's disease). Muscle & Nerve. 2007;**36**:816-820

[78] Nolano M, Provitera V, Crisci C, Saltalamacchia AM, Wendelschafer-Crabb G, Kennedy WR, et al. Small fibers involvement in Friedreich's ataxia. Annals of Neurology. 2001;**50**: 17-25

[79] Ren Y, Liu W, Li Y, Sun B, Li Y, Yang F, et al. Cutaneous somatic and autonomic nerve TDP-43 deposition in amyotrophic lateral sclerosis. Journal of Neurology. 2018;**265**:1753-1763

[80] Symons FJ, Wendelschafer-Crabb G, Kennedy W, Hardrict R, Dahl N, Bodfish JW. Evidence of aletered epidermal nerve fiber morphology in adults with self-injurious behaviour and neurodevelopmental disorders. Pain. 2008;**134**:232-237

[81] Taylor SW, Laughlin RS, Kumar N, Goodman B, Klein CJ, Dyck PJ, et al. Clinical, physiological and pathological characterisation of the sensory predominant peripheral neuropathy in copper deficiency. Journal of Neurology, Neurosurgery, and Psychiatry. 2017;**88**:839-845

[82] Kennedy WR, Selim MM, Brink TS, Hodges JS, Wendelschafer-Crabb G, Foster SX, et al. A new device to quantify tactile sensation in neuropathy. Neurology. 2011;**76**:1642-1649

[83] Verendeev A, Thomas C, McFarlin SC, Hopkins WD, Phillips KA, Sherwood CC. Comparative analysis of Meissner's corpuscles in the fingertips of primates. Journal of Anatomy. 2015;**227**: 72-80

[84] Li J, Bai Y, Ghandour K, Qin P, Grandis M, Trostinskaia A, et al. Skin biopsies in myelin-related neuropathies: Bringing molecular pathology to the bedside. Brain. 2005;**128**:1168-1177

[85] Terracciano C, Pachatz C, Rastelli E, Pastore FS, Melone MAB, Massa R. Neurofibromatous neuropathy: An ultrastructural study. Ultrastructural Pathology. 2018;**42**:312-316

[86] Devigili G, De Filippo M, Ciana G, Dardis A, Lettieri C, Rinaldo S, et al. Chronic pain in Gaucher disease: Skeletal or neuropathic origin? Orphanet Journal of Rare Diseases. 2017; **12**:148

Section 2

Etiologies and Pathogenesis

Chapter 2

HIV-Associated Sensory Neuropathy

Fitri Octaviana, Ahmad Yanuar Safri, Darma Imran and Patricia Price

Abstract

As advances in the treatment of HIV are now allowing patients a longer life span, further comorbidities become apparent. This includes sensory neuropathy (HIV-SN) which can affect a patient's quality of life. Here, we review factors influencing HIV-SN in patients receiving antiretroviral therapy that promotes this condition and in the modern era when these therapies have been withdrawn. This has halved the incidence of HIV-SN, but the condition remains significant in the lives of many sufferers. Genetic polymorphisms that influence pathogenesis of HIV-SN have indicated likely mechanisms, but studies of skin biopsies and animal models are needed to confirm the roles of the encoded proteins.

Keywords: HIV sensory neuropathy, inflammation, neuronal repair

1. Introduction

Management of HIV patients is now focused on their quality of life as antiretroviral therapy (ART) increases life expectancy. However, with longer lives, a growing number of patients experience a neurological disorder that predominantly affects small fibers. HIV-associated sensory neuropathy (HIV-SN) may arise not only as a result of HIV infection itself but also as a side effect of ART. The clinical pictures triggered by HIV infection or ART are very similar and include neuropathic pain, tingling sensation, and numbness [1–3]. HIV-SN is one of the most common complications of HIV infection.

The incidence and prevalence of HIV-SN vary widely—perhaps because most studies do not distinguish between neuropathy due to HIV itself and due to ART regimens with different risk profiles. Cross-sectional studies including patients receiving ART identify HIV-SN in 16–50% of HIV patients [4–6]. ART that includes the non-nucleotide reverse transcriptase inhibitor (NNRTI), stavudine (d4T), is associated with high prevalence of HIV-SN. The prevalence in Melbourne was up to 42%, whereas in Kuala Lumpur and Jakarta, the reported level was lower, 19 and 34%, respectively [7]. Stavudine is no longer in first-line therapy, and the prevalence of HIV-SN is almost halved (14.2%) compared to data from the same clinic in Indonesia when patients received stavudine [8].

In untreated patients, the risk factors for HIV-SN were severe HIV disease marked by low numbers of $CD4^+$ T cells and high viral loads (HIV RNA) in plasma. In the era of ART (including stavudine), the risk factors of HIV-SN included older age, height, <50 $CD4^+$ T cells/mm^3, malnutrition, and concurrent diabetes [1, 7, 9, 10]. HIV-SN was also more common in African-Americans [3] and Hispanics [11]. Genetic polymorphisms may alter risk for HIV-SN in Africans [12–14], Asians [15], and Caucasians [16]. These factors are discussed in more detail here.

2. Clinical features and diagnostic criteria

There are two forms of HIV-SN—distal symmetrical polyneuropathy in HIV (DSP) and antiretroviral toxic neuropathy (ATN). DSP arises at later stages of HIV infection, while ATN is caused by neurotoxic effects of antiretroviral drugs [10, 17]. These two forms cannot be distinguished clinically, so they are grouped as HIV-SN when seen in patients receiving ART.

The most frequent symptoms of HIV-SN are pain, numbness, and burning sensations. The symptoms can be progressive, predominantly affecting the soles of the feet and may become more severe at night. Physical examination may reveal hyperalgesia and allodynia, with absent physiological reflexes and sensory loss in the distal limb segments, including sensitivity to vibration [1, 9–11]. Clinical symptoms usually occur first on the lower limbs for several months but may spread upward. Since HIV-SN predominantly affects small nerve fibers, the clinical signs can also manifest as autonomic neuropathy with postural hypotension and urinary dysfunction [18]. Guidelines for the diagnosis and management of HIV-SN are available [e.g., https://www.hiv.va.gov/provider/manual-primary-care/peripheral-neuropathy.asp] but require adaptation to accommodate differences between patient populations, structures of medical care, and available resources.

Perhaps, the optimal tool to screen HIV-SN is AIDS Clinical Trial Group Brief Peripheral Neuropathy Screening Test (ACTG BPNST). This test has been used in many countries including Australia, the USA, India, South Africa, and Indonesia. It is relatively inexpensive, is fairly easy to do, and takes less than 10 minutes to perform but has low sensitivity. A study comparing BPNST to modified Total Neuropathy Scores (mTNS) in HIV patients on ART (including d4T, ddI, ddC) found that the sensitivity of BPNST was 49%, whereas the specificity was high at 88% [17]. Peripheral neuropathy can be diagnosed if there is ≥1 symptom assessed in the BPNST list and one of the following signs: decreased Achilles reflexes or decreased sensibility to vibration when a tuning fork is held on a toe. This definition means that patients with two abnormal signs but no symptoms are not considered to have HIV-SN. This may contribute to variations in the prevalence of peripheral neuropathy in HIV reported in various studies. Some studies consider this intermediate group as asymptomatic peripheral neuropathy with the assumption that they can become symptomatic in time. Ellis et al. defined peripheral neuropathy as a decrease in Achilles tendon reflexes or decreased perception of vibration in both legs. The sensitivity increased by 80% but the specificity decreased to 59% [19].

Clinically, peripheral neuropathy can also be classified as small- or large-fiber neuropathy. The latter manifests as the loss of joint position and vibration sense and sensory ataxia, whereas small-fiber neuropathy manifests as neuropathic pain, impairment of temperature sensing, and autonomic function. A nerve conduction study (NCS) can include sensory and motor nerve conduction and help in documenting sensory motor deficits that mainly affect large-fiber nerves [20]. As HIV-SN is a predominately small-fiber neuropathy, NCS is often normal [21]. In HIV-SN patients, ATN- and HIV-associated DSP often cannot be distinguished since patients can have both types at same time. However, there are some evidences that ATN primarily impairs small-fiber nerves, whereas HIV-associated neuropathy (DSP) has been linked to large-fiber nerves [22, 23].

Stimulated skin wrinkling (SSW) test is a method to assess small nerve fiber function using exposure to eutectic mixture of local anesthetic. It has been shown to correlate with intraepidermal nerve fiber density (IENFD) in patients with a sensory neuropathy [24] and has high sensitivity compared to other assessments of small-fiber neuropathy in diabetic patients [25]. Skin wrinkling occurs as a result of vasoconstriction in the glabrous skin, mediated by postganglionic sympathetic fibers [26]. Other assessments that have been used to detect small-fiber neuropathy in HIV-SN patients include quantitative sudomotor axon reflex tests (QSART) [27], quantitative sensory tests (QST) [18], and sympathetic skin responses (SSR) [22, 23].

Skin biopsies are the gold standard for the detection of damage to small-diameter sensory nerves, including non-myelinated and myelinated intraepidermal nerve fibers. Lower nerve fiber densities have been demonstrated in patients with HIV-SN [18]. Studies have used several different techniques. The European Federation of Neurological Societies recommended a biopsy of the skin to a depth of 3 mm by using a skin punch biopsy on the distal limbs to calculate the linear density or nerve fibers with a minimum of 50 µm-thick slices, fixed in a 2% solution of paraformaldehyde-lysine-periodate (2% PLP). Immunohistochemical staining techniques recommended are bright-field immunohistochemistry and indirect immunofluorescence [28]. PGP9.5 immunofluorescence allows nerves to be visualized using a confocal microscope [29]. Smaller intraepidermal nerve fiber densities (IENFD) in HIV-SN patients correlated with the clinical and electrophysiological severity [30]. Skin biopsies can also be used to identify cells and mediators that contribute to SN. These are discussed later in this chapter.

3. Clinical factors influence the risk of HIV-SN

Analyses of the risk factor of HIV-SN require that we consider the condition in three distinct eras—(1) pre-ART, (2) the use of combination ART that included stavudine (d4T), and (3) the use of non-neurotoxic ART. In the pre-ART era, the risk factors for developing HIV-SN included HIV disease severity, low $CD4^+$ T-cell counts, high viral load, and older age [31, 32]. In the second era, the risk factors are older age, height, low nadir $CD4^+$ T-cell counts, HIV duration, malnutrition, diabetes mellitus, dyslipidemia, and the use of neurotoxic drugs (usually stavudine; see **Table 1**; [7, 14, 15, 33, 34]). Stavudine is no longer recommended by the WHO as first-line ART and is now rarely used anywhere in the world, but HIV-SN has

Demographic risk factors	Genetic risk factors
Low nadir $CD4^+$ T-cell count HIV duration Age Height High plasma HIV RNA Diabetes mellitus Malnutrition Neurotoxic drugs • NRTI: stavudine, didanosine • Protease inhibitors: indinavir, ritonavir, saquinavir	Race (more common in African populations) Polymorphisms in • Mitochondrial DNA (mtDNA) • *HFE* (affecting iron metabolism) • Cytokine genes (*IL4, IL10, IL12B*) • *TNF* gene block (central MHC) • *P2X4R, P2X7R* (purinergic receptors) • *CAMKK2* (affecting neuronal repair)

Table 1.
Genetic and demographic risk factors affecting HIV-SN in patients receiving ART.

not disappeared. The risk factors of HIV-SN in patients on ART without stavudine are almost the same as in the pre-ART era—high plasma viral load and older age [8]. Isoniazid is widely used as therapy for tuberculosis and has been recognized as a risk factor for neuropathy for a long time. It remains weakly associated with HIV-SN even though patients receiving isoniazid are also given B6 supplementation to prevent neuropathy. Protease inhibitor (PI) exposure may be a risk factor of HIV-SN. Lopinavir, indinavir, and ritonavir, but not nelfinavir, were associated with neuropathy in one study [35].

4. Genetic risk factors

The risk of HIV-SN cannot be correlated with a single genetic variant, so candidate genes are discussed separately (see **Table 1**). It is of interest to determine if any aligns with the greater sensitivity of individuals of African descent [13, 14, 36].

4.1 Genes in linkage disequilibrium with TNF or encoding components of pathways regulated by TNF

In patients receiving stavudine, haplotypic combinations of alleles of single-nucleotide polymorphisms (SNP) spanning the tumor necrosis factor (TNF) block in the central major histocompatibility complex (MHC) associate with variations in the prevalence of HIV-SN, but the associations were different in Africans and Asians [12]. For example, a polymorphism in intron 10 of BAT1 (marking an MHC haplotype associated with several inflammatory disorders) and a polymorphism in the promoter region of the *TNFA* gene (TNF-1031) were associated with an increased risk of HIV-SN in Caucasians [37]. TNF-1031*2 is associated with an increased risk of HIV-SN in Indonesian HIV-positive patients who receive stavudine [15, 16]. However, in Africans, different SNP alleles were found in linkage disequilibrium with TNF-1031*2, so TNF-1031*2 was not associated with HIV-SN. These findings link HIV-SN with an unknown SNP in the TNF block marked by (but distinct from) TNF-1031. The link between HIV-SN and inflammation was supported by studies linking *IL4* genotypes with HIV-SN in Africans receiving stavudine [13].

4.2 The *P2X7R*, *P2X4R*, and *CAMKK2* gene cluster: Inflammation and neuronal repair

Goullee et al. linked SNP in three genes *P2X7R*, *P2X4R*, and *CAMKK2* with HIV-SN in African patients treated with stavudine. In a logistic regression model which included demographic analyses, SNP in *CAMKK2*, and to a lesser extent *P2X7R* and *P2X4R*, demonstrated independent associations with HIV-SN ($p < 0.0001$; $R^2 = 0.19$) [14].

The P2X7R receptor is expressed by microglia and may be involved in neuropathic pain, as its ablation or inhibition in animal models of neuropathy can reduce responses to painful stimuli [38]. Conversely, stimulation of P2X7R will increase the release of pro-inflammatory cytokines such as IL-1β, IL-6, and TNFα [39] as well as pro-inflammatory chemokines such as CXCL2 and CCL3, which have been implicated in neuropathic pain [40, 41].

In animal studies, P2X4R was activated in spinal microglial cells in rats with induced pain [42]. Mice with disrupted *P2X4R* genes showed reduced pain response in two models of chronic pain (inflammatory and neuropathic) [43]. P2X4R is upregulated after peripheral nerve injury which results in increased activity of mitogen p38 [44]. This process initiates the release of brain-derived neurotropic factor (BDNF). BDNF induces neuronal hyperexcitability through interaction with the TrkB receptor [45, 46].

The *CAMKK2* gene encodes calcium-/calmodulin-dependent protein kinase 2 (CaMKK2), which acts as a pervasive second messenger of Ca^{2+} in many cellular functions such as energy balance, neuronal differentiation, and inflammation [47]. CaMKK2 plays a role in neural plasticity and neurite growth by activating another protein kinase CaMKI [48]. *CAMKK2* and *P2X4R* polymorphisms affect TNFα production in vitro. This suggests a mechanism for their impact on HIV-SN [49]. Hence, polymorphisms in *CAMKK2* may affect inflammation or neuronal growth.

4.3 Mitochondrial haplotypes and iron metabolism

The process of mitochondrial toxicity induced by ART is not a simple drug toxicity, but mitochondrial DNA (mtDNA) SNP has a role in developing HIV-SN in patients receiving NRTI. SNP in African mtDNA haplogroup L1c and European haplogroup J is associated with decreased prevalence of HIV-SN compared with all other haplogroups [36]. Moreover, Thai persons belonging to mtDNA haplogroup B were more likely to develop HIV-SN [50].

HIV-1 *Nef* protein may influence iron levels via interactions with the hemochromatosis protein HFE in humans [51]. In an observational prospective study, Kallianpur et al. suggested that disruption of iron homeostasis due to HIV infection might damage neurons and potentially lead to HIV-SN. They presented evidence that the *HFE* C282Y mutation may be a protective factor in HIV patients using NRTI [52]. They subsequently linked polymorphisms in iron management genes with increased risk (*TF, CP, ACO1, BMP6, B2M*) and reduced risk (*TF, TFRC, BMP6, ACO1, SLC11A2, FXN*) of HIV-SN [53].

5. The pathophysiology of HIV-SN

The pathophysiology of HIV-SN is not completely understood, but there are several promising theories. It remains unclear whether HIV inflicts direct damage in the nerve body of dorsal root ganglia (DRG) or damages nerve fibers; both will lead to the development of distal axonopathies. HIV causes distal axon degeneration, reduction of nerve fiber in DRG, infiltration of inflammation cells, and reduction of the intraepidermal nerve fiber (IENFD) count [2]. As HIV itself cannot directly infect nerve bodies, destruction of neuron in HIV-SN may be caused by neurotoxic agents released by activated macrophage and satellite glial cells (TNF-α, IL-1β, chemokines), viral proteins with neurotoxic properties (gp41, gp120, Tat, Vpr), infection of perineural cells, or combinations of these processes [54–58]. A study in simian immunodeficiency virus macaque model confirmed that HIV infection activates perineuronal inflammatory cells (including macrophages and lymphocytes) in trigeminal ganglia and DRG during the early stage of infection. In the later stage, neuronal damage becomes evident, and regenerative capacity of small epidermal nerve is impaired [59].

HIV infection may cause macrophages to respond to the axonal degeneration (even in mild cases) causing inflammation of the nerves and DRG. Pro-inflammatory mediators were released by Schwann cells at DRG and may accumulate adjacent to peripheral nerves, activate apoptotic pathways and cause damage to the nerves directly or indirectly (reviewed in [55]). The gp120 virus protein may act directly on chemokine receptors expressed on neurons and cause pain [60]. A histopathology study of skin biopsies from HIV-SN patients on ART without stavudine confirmed the presence of inflammatory macrophages and T cells expressing some chemokine receptors (CX3CR1, CCR2, CCR5), along with reduced IENFD [61].

HIV protein gp120 is a component of the viral glycoprotein sheath. The entry of the HIV virus into cells requires the interaction of gp120 with CD4 glycoprotein and a chemokine receptor (usually CXCR4 and/or CCR5) which may be expressed on neurons or infiltrating inflammatory cells. Several chemokine receptors, such as CCR2, CCR5, and CXCR4, and CX_3CR1 (fractalkine receptor) are located in primary afferent neurons or secondary neurons of the spinal dorsal horn. Chemokines and gp120 can cause pain through direct effects on chemokine receptors expressed by nociceptive neurons [62]. For example, binding of gp120 to CXCR4 receptors increases the release of CCL5, which binds CCR5 and triggers the release of TNFα and other neurotoxic substances. These interactions activate an influx of Ca^{2+}, kinase cascades, and STAT3 signaling leading to the signs and symptoms of HIV-SN. The pathways have been reviewed previously [61, 63].

The pathophysiology of HIV-SN in patients on stavudine may reflect damage to the mitochondria of neurons and axons via damage to mitochondrial DNA (mtDNA) [64]. Inhibition of mtDNA gamma polymerase, mtDNA intercalation, and damage in stress response of mitochondria has been demonstrated in vitro in cultures of T-lymphoblastoid cells [65]. This finding is further supported by differences in haplotypes or SNP in mtDNA in Europeans, Hispanics, and Africans that may contribute to differences in the prevalence of HIV-SN [36, 52, 66, 67].

6. Therapeutic options

Management of HIV-SN aims to avoid further nerve damage and minimize the patients' symptoms especially neuropathic pain. Some studies showed that smoked cannabis is effective and has analgesic value to relieve pain in HIV-SN patients [68, 69]. However, due to legal issues in many countries, the recommendation of smoked cannabis has been controversial. Other pharmacological treatments recommended for neuropathic pain are amitriptyline, pregabalin, and gabapentin [70]. However, these medications were not superior to the placebo in HIV-SN patients [71–73]. Another option is non-pharmacological treatment such as acupuncture and hypnosis. However, acupuncture was not superior to the placebo to improve pain in HIV patients [74]. A small study showed that hypnosis showed benefit to reduce the pain score in HIV-SN patients [75].

7. Conclusions and future directions

Despite the withdrawal of the most toxic drugs from recommended ART regimens, HIV-SN remains a common neurological complication of HIV disease. The risk factors of HIV-SN have changed with changes in ART from the patient's age and height to the efficacy of ART and the use of protease inhibitors. Genetic polymorphisms that influence pathogenesis of HIV-SN will provide candidate molecules, which may contribute to pathogenesis, but studies of skin biopsies from patients are needed to confirm the roles of the encoded proteins. Animal models may reveal mechanisms for neuropathy and pain by HIV proteins but do not mimic the complexities of HIV disease in patients.

Author details

Fitri Octaviana[1,2*], Ahmad Yanuar Safri[1,2], Darma Imran[1,2] and Patricia Price[1,3,4]

1 Neurology Department, Faculty of Medicine, Universitas Indonesia, Jakarta, Indonesia

2 Neurology Department, Cipto Mangunkusumo Hospital, Jakarta, Indonesia

3 School of Biomedical Sciences, Curtin University, Bentley, Australia

4 School of Physiology, University of Witwatersrand, Johannesburg, South Africa

*Address all correspondence to: fitri.octaviana@gmail.com

References

[1] Pardo CA, McArthur JC, Griffin JW. HIV neuropathy: Insights in the pathology of HIV peripheral nerve disease. Journal of the Peripheral Nervous System. 2001;**6**:21-27

[2] Schütz SG, Robinson-Papp J. HIV-related neuropathy: Current perspectives. HIV AIDS. 2013;**5**:243-251

[3] Anziska Y, Helzner EP, Crystal H, Glesby MJ, Plankey M, Weber K, et al. The relationship between race and HIV-distal sensory polyneuropathy in a large cohort of US women. Journal of the Neurological Sciences. 2012;**315**:129-132

[4] Morgello S. HIV-associated distal sensory polyneuropathy in the era of highly active antiretroviral therapy: The Manhattan HIV Brain Bank. Archives of Neurology. 2004;**61**:546-551

[5] Dubey TN, Raghuvanshi SS, Sharma H, Saxena R. HIV neuropathy in pre-HAART patients and it's correlation with risk factors in Central India. Neurology India. 2013;**61**:478-480

[6] Centner CM, Little F, Van, Der Watt JJ, Vermaak J-R, Dave JA, Levitt NS, et al. Evolution of sensory neuropathy after initiation of antiretroviral therapy: HIV-DSP evolution on ART. Muscle & Nerve. 2018;**57**:371-379

[7] Cherry CL, Affandi JS, Imran D, Yunihastuti E, Smyth K, Vanar S, et al. Age and height predict neuropathy risk in patients with HIV prescribed stavudine. Neurology. 2009;**73**:315-320

[8] Octaviana F, Safri AY, Setiawan DD, Estiasari R, Imran D, Ranakusuma T, et al. Detectable plasma HIV RNA is associated with sensory neuropathy in HIV patients treated without stavudine. Journal of Acquired Immune Deficiency Syndromes. 2018. publish ahead of print. DOI: 10.1097/QAI.0000000000001836

[9] Gonzalez-Duarte A, Robinson-Papp J, Simpson DM. Diagnosis and management of HIV-associated neuropathy. Neurologic Clinics. 2008;**26**:821-832

[10] Centner CM, Bateman KJ, Heckmann JM. Manifestations of HIV infection in the peripheral nervous system. Lancet Neurology. 2013;**12**:295-309

[11] Robinson-Papp J, Gonzalez-Duarte A, Simpson DM, Rivera-Mindt M, Morgello S. The roles of ethnicity and antiretrovirals in HIV-associated polyneuropathy: A pilot study. Journal of Acquired Immune Deficiency Syndromes. 2009;**51**:569-573

[12] Wadley AL, Hendry LM, Kamerman PR, Chew CS, Price P, Cherry CL, et al. Role of TNF block genetic variants in HIV-associated sensory neuropathy in black southern Africans. European Journal of Human Genetics. 2015;**23**:363-368

[13] Wadley AL, Kamerman PR, Chew CSN, Lombard Z, Cherry CL, Price P. A polymorphism in IL4 may associate with sensory neuropathy in African HIV patients. Molecular Immunology. 2013;**55**:197-199

[14] Goullee H, Wadley AL, Cherry CL, Allcock RJN, Black M, Kamerman PR, et al. Polymorphisms in CAMKK2 may predict sensory neuropathy in African HIV patients. Journal of Neurovirology. 2016;**22**:508-517

[15] Affandi JS, Price P, Imran D, Yunihastuti E, Djauzi S, Cherry CL. Can we predict neuropathy risk before stavudine prescription in a resource-limited setting? AIDS Research and Human Retroviruses. 2008;**24**:1281-1284

[16] Chew CSN, Cherry CL, Imran D, Yunihastuti E, Kamarulzaman A, Varna S, et al. Tumour necrosis

factor haplotypes associated with sensory neuropathy in Asian and Caucasian human immunodeficiency virus patients. Tissue Antigens. 2011;**77**:126-130

[17] Hahn K, Husstedt I. HIV associated neuropathies. In: HIV Infection in the Era of Highly Active Antiretroviral Treatment and Some of Its Association [Internet]. IntechOpen; 2011 [cited 2018 Jun 5]. p. 15. Available from: https://www.intechopen.com/books/hiv-infection-in-the-era-of-highly-active-antiretroviral-treatment-and-some-of-its-associated-complications

[18] Phillips TJC, Brown M, Ramirez JD, Perkins J, Woldeamanuel YW, Williams AC de C, et al. Sensory, psychological, and metabolic dysfunction in HIV-associated peripheral neuropathy: A cross-sectional deep profiling study. Pain. 2014;**155**:1846-1860

[19] Ellis RJ, Evans SR, Clifford DB, Moo LR, McArthur JC, Collier AC, et al. Clinical validation of the NeuroScreen. Journal of Neurovirology. 2005;**11**:503-511

[20] Misra UK, Kalita J, Nair PP. Diagnostic approach to peripheral neuropathy. Annals of Indian Academy of Neurology. 2008;**11**:89-97

[21] Brew BJ. The peripheral nerve complications of human immunodeficiency virus (HIV) infection. Muscle & Nerve. 2003;**28**:542-552

[22] Kokotis P, Schmelz M, Skopelitis EE, Kordossis T, Karandreas N. Differential sensitivity of thick and thin fibers to HIV and therapy-induced neuropathy. Autonomic Neuroscience. 2007;**136**:90-95

[23] Kokotis P, Schmelz M, Papadimas GK, Skopelitis EE, Aroni K, Kordossis T, et al. Polyneuropathy induced by HIV disease and antiretroviral therapy. Clinical Neurophysiology. 2013;**124**:176-182

[24] Teoh HL, Chow A, Wilder-Smith E. Skin wrinkling for diagnosing small fibre neuropathy: Comparison with epidermal nerve density and sympathetic skin response. Journal of Neurology, Neurosurgery, and Psychiatry. 2008;**79**:835-837

[25] Ping Ng KW, Ong JJY, Nyein Nyein TD, Liang S, Chan YC, Lee KO, et al. EMLA-induced skin wrinkling for the detection of diabetic neuropathy. Frontiers in Neurology. 2013;**4**:1-7

[26] Wilder-Smith E, Chow A. Water immersion and EMLA cause similar digit skin wrinkling and vasoconstriction. Microvascular Research. 2003;**66**:68-72

[27] Boger MS, Hulgan T, Haas DW, Mitchell V, Smith AG, Singleton JR, et al. Measures of small-fiber neuropathy in HIV infection. Autonomic Neuroscience. 2012;**169**:56-61

[28] Lauria G, Cornblath DR, Johansson O, McArthur JC, Mellgren SI, Nolano M, et al. EFNS guidelines on the use of skin biopsy in the diagnosis of peripheral neuropathy. European Journal of Neurology. 2005;**12**:747-758

[29] Van Acker N, Ragé M, Sluydts E, Knaapen MWM, De Bie M, Timmers M, et al. Automated PGP9.5 immunofluorescence staining: A valuable tool in the assessment of small fiber neuropathy? BMC Research Notes. 2016;**9**:280-290

[30] Zhou L, Kitch DW, Evans SR, Hauer P, Raman S, Ebenezer GJ, et al. Correlates of epidermal nerve fiber densities in HIV-associated distal sensory polyneuropathy. Neurology. 2007;**68**:2113-2119

[31] Childs EA, Lyles RH, Selnes OA, Chen B, Miller EN, Cohen BA, et al. Plasma viral load and CD4 lymphocytes predict HIV-associated dementia and sensory neuropathy. Neurology. 1999;**52**:607-613

[32] Tagliati M, Grinnell J, Godbold J, Simpson DM. Peripheral nerve function in HIV infection. Archives of Neurology. 1999;**56**:84-89

[33] Evans SR, Ellis RJ, Chen H, Yeh T, Lee AJ, Schifitto G, et al. Peripheral neuropathy in HIV: Prevalence and risk factors. AIDS. 2011;**25**:919-928

[34] Nakamoto BK, McMurtray A, Davis J, Valcour V, Watters MR, Shiramizu B, et al. Incident neuropathy in HIV-infected patients on HAART. AIDS Research and Human Retroviruses. 2010;**26**:759-765

[35] Pettersen JA, Jones G, Worthington C, Krentz HB, Keppler OT, Hoke A, et al. Sensory neuropathy in human immunodeficiency virus/acquired immunodeficiency syndrome patients: Protease inhibitor–mediated neurotoxicity. Annals of Neurology. 2006;**59**:816-824

[36] Holzinger ER, Hulgan T, Ellis RJ, Samuels DC, Ritchie MD, Haas DW, et al. Mitochondrial DNA variation and HIV-associated sensory neuropathy in CHARTER. Journal of Neurovirology. 2012;**18**:511-520

[37] Cherry CL, Rosenow A, Affandi JS, McArthur JC, Wesselingh SL, Price P. Cytokine genotype suggests a role for inflammation in nucleoside analog-associated sensory neuropathy (NRTI-SN) and predicts an individual's NRTI-SN risk. AIDS Research and Human Retroviruses. 2008;**24**:117-123

[38] Makoto T, Hidetoshi T-S, Kazuhide I. P2X4R and P2X7R in neuropathic pain. WIREs Membrane Transport and Signaling. 2012;**1**:513-521

[39] Kawasaki Y, Zhang L, Cheng J-K, Ji R-R. Cytokine mechanisms of central sensitization: Distinct and overlapping role of interleukin-1beta, interleukin-6, and tumor necrosis factor-alpha in regulating synaptic and neuronal activity in the superficial spinal cord. The Journal of Neuroscience. 2008;**28**:5189-5194

[40] Kataoka A, Tozaki-Saitoh H, Koga Y, Tsuda M, Inoue K. Activation of P2X7 receptors induces CCL3 production in microglial cells through transcription factor NFAT. Journal of Neurochemistry. 2009;**108**:115-125

[41] Shiratori M, Tozaki-Saitoh H, Yoshitake M, Tsuda M, Inoue K. P2X7 receptor activation induces CXCL2 production in microglia through NFAT and PKC/MAPK pathways. Journal of Neurochemistry. 2010;**114**:810-819

[42] Guo L-H, Trautmann K, Schluesener HJ. Expression of P2X4 receptor by lesional activated microglia during formalin-induced inflammatory pain. Journal of Neuroimmunology. 2005;**163**:120-127

[43] Tsuda M, Kuboyama K, Inoue T, Nagata K, Tozaki-Saitoh H, Inoue K. Behavioral phenotypes of mice lacking purinergic P2X4 receptors in acute and chronic pain assays. Molecular Pain. 2009;**5**:28-34

[44] Tsuda M, Masuda T, Tozaki-Saitoh H, Inoue K. P2X4 receptors and neuropathic pain. Frontiers in Cellular Neuroscience. 2013;**7**:191

[45] Toulme E, Khakh BS. Imaging P2X4 receptor lateral mobility in microglia: Regulation by calcium and p38 MAPK. The Journal of Biological Chemistry. 2012;**287**:14734-14748

[46] Trang T, Beggs S, Wan X, Salter MW. P2X4-receptor-mediated synthesis and release of brain-derived neurotrophic factor in microglia is dependent on calcium and p38-mitogen-activated protein kinase activation. The Journal of Neuroscience. 2009;**29**:3518-3528

[47] Zhang X, Guo L, Collage RD, Stripay JL, Tsung A, Lee JS, et al.

Calcium/calmodulin-dependent protein kinase (CaMK) Ialpha mediates the macrophage inflammatory response to sepsis. Journal of Leukocyte Biology. 2011;**90**:249-261

[48] Wayman GA, Lee Y-S, Tokumitsu H, Silva AJ, Soderling TR. Calmodulin-kinases: Modulators of neuronal development and plasticity. Neuron. 2008;**59**:914-931

[49] Gaff J, Halstrom S, Temple SEL, Baltic S, Kamerman P, Price P. Polymorphisms in P2X4R and CAMKK2 may affect TNFα production: Implications for a role in HIV-associated sensory neuropathy. Human Immunology. 2018;**79**:224-227

[50] Hulgan T, Levinson RT, Gerschenson M, Phanuphak N, Ananworanich J, Teeratakulpisarm N, et al. Epidermal nerve fiber density, oxidative stress, and mitochondrial haplogroups in HIV-infected Thais initiating therapy. AIDS. 2014;**28**:1625-1633

[51] Drakesmith H, Chen N, Ledermann H, Screaton G, Townsend A, Xu X-N. HIV-1 Nef down-regulates the hemochromatosis protein HFE, manipulating cellular iron homeostasis. Proceedings of the National Academy of Sciences of the United States of America. 2005;**102**:11017-11022

[52] Kallianpur AR, Hulgan T, Canter JA, Ritchie MD, Haines JL, Robbins GK, et al. Hemochromatosis (HFE) gene mutations and peripheral neuropathy during antiretroviral therapy. AIDS. 2006;**20**:1503-1513

[53] Kallianpur AR, Jia P, Ellis RJ, Zhao Z, Bloss C, Wen W, et al. Genetic variation in iron metabolism is associated with neuropathic pain and pain severity in HIV-infected patients on antiretroviral therapy. PLoS One. 2014;**9**:e103123

[54] Abbadie C, Bhangoo S, De YK, Malcangio M, Melik-Parsadaniantz S, White FA. Chemokines and pain mechanisms. Brain Research Reviews. 2009;**60**:125-134

[55] Kamerman PR, Moss PJ, Weber J, Wallace VCJ, Rice ASC, Huang W. Pathogenesis of HIV-associated sensory neuropathy: Evidence from in vivo and in vitro experimental models. Journal of the Peripheral Nervous System. 2012;**17**:19-31

[56] Acharjee S, Noorbakhsh F, Stemkowski PL, Olechowski C, Cohen EA, Ballanyi K, et al. HIV-1 viral protein R causes peripheral nervous system injury associated with in vivo neuropathic pain. The FASEB Journal. 2010;**24**:4343-4353

[57] Melli G, Keswani SC, Fischer A, Chen W, Höke A. Spatially distinct and functionally independent mechanisms of axonal degeneration in a model of HIV-associated sensory neuropathy. Brain. 2006;**129**:1330-1338

[58] Hahn K, Robinson B, Anderson C, Li W, Pardo CA, Morgello S, et al. Differential effects of HIV infected macrophages on dorsal root ganglia neurons and axons. Experimental Neurology. 2008;**210**:30-40

[59] Mangus LM, Dorsey JL, Laast VA, Ringkamp M, Ebenezer GJ, Hauer P, et al. Unraveling the pathogenesis of HIV peripheral neuropathy: Insights from a simian immunodeficiency virus macaque model. ILAR Journal. 2014;**54**:296-303

[60] Hao S. The molecular and pharmacological mechanisms of HIV-related neuropathic pain. Current Neuropharmacology. 2013;**11**:499-512

[61] Mountford J, Octaviana F, Estiasari R, Setiawan DD, Ariyanto I, Lee S, et al. Ex vivo expression of chemokine receptors on cells surrounding

cutaneous nerves in patients with HIV-associated sensory neuropathy. AIDS. 2018;**32**:431-441

[62] Oh SB, Tran PB, Gillard SE, Hurley RW, Hammond DL, Miller RJ. Chemokines and glycoprotein120 produce pain hypersensitivity by directly exciting primary nociceptive neurons. The Journal of Neuroscience. 2001;**21**:5027-5035

[63] Kiguchi N, Kobayashi Y, Kishioka S. Chemokines and cytokines in neuroinflammation leading to neuropathic pain. Current Opinion in Pharmacology. 2012;**12**:55-61

[64] Lehmann HC, Chen W, Borzan J, Mankowski JL, Höke A. Mitochondrial dysfunction in distal axons contributes to human immunodeficiency virus sensory neuropathy. Annals of Neurology. 2011;**69**:100-110

[65] Höschele D. Cell culture models for the investigation of NRTI-induced mitochondrial toxicity. Toxicology In Vitro. 2006;**20**:535-546

[66] Canter JA, Haas DW, Kallianpur AR, Ritchie MD, Robbins GK, Shafer RW, et al. The mitochondrial pharmacogenomics of haplogroup T: MTND2*LHON4917G and antiretroviral therapy-associated peripheral neuropathy. The Pharmacogenomics Journal. 2008;**8**:71-77

[67] Canter JA, Robbins GK, Selph D, Clifford DB, Kallianpur AR, Shafer R, et al. African mitochondrial DNA subhaplogroups and peripheral neuropathy during antiretroviral therapy. The Journal of Infectious Diseases. 2010;**201**:1703-1707

[68] Abrams DI, Jay CA, Shade SB, Vizoso H, Reda H, Press S, et al. Cannabis in painful HIV-associated sensory neuropathy: A randomized placebo-controlled trial. Neurology. 2007;**68**:515-521

[69] Ellis RJ, Toperoff W, Vaida F, Van Den Brande G, Gonzales J, Gouaux B, et al. Smoked medicinal cannabis for neuropathic pain in HIV: A randomized, crossover clinical trial. Neuropsychopharmacology. 2009;**34**:672-680

[70] Finnerup NB, Attal N, Haroutounian S, McNicol E, Baron R, Dworkin RH, et al. Pharmacotherapy for neuropathic pain in adults: A systematic review and meta-analysis. Lancet Neurology. 2015;**14**:162-173

[71] Kieburtz K, Simpson D, Yiannoutsos C, Max M, Hall C, Ellis RJ, et al. A randomized trial of amitriptyline and mexiletine for painful neuropathy in HIV infection. AIDS clinical trial group 242 protocol team. Neurology. 1998;**51**:1682-1688

[72] Simpson DM, Schifitto G, Clifford DB, Murphy TK, Cruz ED-D, Glue P, et al. Pregabalin for painful HIV neuropathy. Neurology. 2010;**74**:413-420

[73] Hahn K, Arendt G, Braun JS, Giesen H-J, Husstedt IW, Maschke M, et al. A placebo-controlled trial of gabapentin for painful HIV-associated sensory neuropathies. Journal of Neurology. 2004;**251**:1260-1266

[74] Shlay JC. Acupuncture and amitriptyline for pain due to HIV-related peripheral neuropathy: A randomized controlled trial. Journal of the American Medical Association. 1998;**280**:1590-1595

[75] Dorfman D, George MC, Schnur J, Simpson DM, Davidson G, Montgomery G. Hypnosis for treatment of HIV neuropathic pain: A preliminary report. Pain Medicine. 2013;**14**:1048-1056

Chapter 3

Peripheral Neuropathy in Connective Tissue Diseases

Mouna Snoussi, Faten Frikha and Zouhir Bahloul

Abstract

Connective tissue diseases are characterized by different organ disorders due to loss of immune system tolerance to autoantigens. Peripheral neuropathy is one of the features of these diseases with variable frequency; it is more prevalent in Sjögren syndrome. Peripheral neuropathy is often seen in the course of the disease. Nonetheless, it may be also a presenting sign or the unique feature of immune system dysfunction. Neuropathies in connective tissue diseases are related mainly to vasculitic disorder. It requires prompt diagnosis and treatment to improve its outcome. Peripheral neuropathy in connective tissue diseases could be multifocal and asymmetric, or confluent and symmetrical. This chapter reviews the clinical, diagnostic and therapeutic features of neuropathies associated with the common diffuse connective tissue diseases.

Keywords: peripheral neuropathy, vasculitis, connective tissue disease, treatment, electromyography, nerve biopsy

1. Introduction

Connective tissue diseases (CTDs) are defined as a group of acquired diseases resulting from persistent immune-mediated inflammation. They are generally the consequence of autoimmune dysregulation resulting in generation of autoreactive T cells or autoantibodies [1]. Immune disorders can affect any organ of the human body responsible for multisystem involvement. The CTDs classily include systemic lupus erythematosus (SLE), Sjögren syndrome (SS), systemic sclerosis (SSc), dermatomyositis and polymyositis (PM/DM), undifferentiated CTD (UTCD) and overlap syndromes such as mixed CTD (MCTD). Most clinicians do not include systemic necrotizing vasculitis, e.g. polyarteritis nodosa, Churg-Strauss syndrome and Wegener's granulomatosis in the category of CTD [1]. Peripheral neuropathies (PN) may complicate many different systemic autoimmune diseases. PN in CTD large clinical, histopathological and pathogenic spectrum [2]. We aim in this chapter to precise the epidemiology, the pathogenesis, the diagnosis and the treatment of neuropathies in CTD including systemic lupus erythematosus (SLE), Sjögren syndrome (SS), dermatomyositis and polymyositis (PM/DM), systemic sclerosis (SSc) and mixed CTD (MCTD).

2. Epidemiology of peripheral neuropathy associated with connective tissue diseases and its topographic distribution

PN is one of the clinical features of CTD with variable frequency and prognosis. It is often seen in the course of the disease. However, it may also be a presenting

IntechOpen

Vasculitic neuropathy
Mononeuropathy multiplex
Asymmetrical polyneuropathy
Distal symmetrical polyneuropathy
Distal axonal polyneuropathy
Compression neuropathy
Sensory neuronopathy
Trigeminal sensory neuropathy
Other types of neuropathies associated with connective tissue disease
Acute demyelinating polyneuropathy
Chronic demyelinating polyneuropathy

Table 1.
Types of neuropathies associated with CTD (adapted from neuropathies in connective tissue disease/Richard K) [12].

sign or the unique feature of immune system dysfunction [3]. The prevalence of PN is different in the literature series depending on the type of CTD and the means of diagnosis. The incidence of PN in SS is 10–60%, and many of these patients (40–93%) present with neuropathy as the sentinel symptom [4]. PN in SLE patients ranges from 25 to 50% based on electrodiagnostic studies. Curiously, the incidence drops to only 5% based on clinical criteria [5, 6]. Finally, PN is rarely associated with the other CTD, namely, SSc, MCTD, DM and PM [4].

PN refers to the part of a spinal nerve distal to the root and plexus. It is a damage or a disease affecting nerves [7–9]. Neuropathy affecting one nerve is called "mononeuropathy" and neuropathy affecting multiple nerves in the same areas on both sides of the body is named "symmetrical polyneuropathy". When separate nerves in disparate areas of the body are affected, the neuropathy is called mononeuritis multiplex, multifocal mononeuropathy or multiple mononeuropathy [8, 10, 11]. Types of neuropathies that are associated with CTD are outlined in **Table 1**.

3. Pathogenesis of peripheral neuropathy in connective tissue diseases

The principal components in the pathogenesis of peripheral nerve lesions in diffuse CTD are ischemia due to vasculitis and immune abnormalities. Generally, most of patients have a combination of the ischemic, immunological and metabolic mechanisms of damage to the peripheral nervous system. Nevertheless, one component may be predominant in a different stage of the disease. In systemic scleroderma, the greater role is played by ischemic mechanisms, mainly in the initial states of the disease, while SLE may involve the participation of immunological mechanisms, especially in acute and subacute disease with high level of autoimmune activity [13].

3.1 Vasculitic neuropathy

The immunopathogenesis of vasculitis in CTD is still unclear. The accumulation of immune complexes in the vasa nervorum initiates the leukocytoclastic reaction, which is characterized by segmental fibrinoid necrosis and transmural inflammatory cell infiltration. Vasculitis induces the occlusion of vasa nervorum at the epineurial arteries and produces nerve infarction. Nerve infarcts typically lead to axonal degeneration [14]. Demyelination and conduction block may occur transiently but are usually not a predominant or persistent finding [15]. The clinical and electrophysiological features of neuropathies correlate with the rapidity of onset of ischemia. Acute ischemia induces the development of mononeuropathy, while prolonged circulatory insufficiency is associated with chronic polyneuropathy. The compression-ischemic mechanism leads to the formation of tunnel syndromes [13, 14, 16, 17]. The Peripheral Nerve Society task force has recently proposed a classification that categorizes vasculitic neuropathy into primary systemic vasculitides, secondary systemic vasculitides including CTD and nonsystemic or localized vasculitis on the basis of disease associations [18].

3.2 Autoimmune disorders

Patients with diffuse CTD may have IgG and IgM anticardiolipin antibodies in their serum, which are associated with severe signs of neural lesions, as demonstrated by electromyogram [13]. Moreover, serum levels of anti-nerve growth factor (NGF) antibodies are greater than normal in 32.1% of patients with diffuse CTD. Increased serum levels of anti-NGF are associated with high disease activity and more severe nervous system involvement [13].

3.3 Metabolic disorder

Peripheral nervous system abnormalities in CTD are also explained by metabolic disorder secondary to aggressive therapy, multiorgan pathology and endocrine abnormalities in these patients. Metabolic disorder may induce a reaction of demyelization and axon dystrophy in severe cases [13].

4. Clinical practice guidelines of peripheral neuropathy in CTD

In CTD neuropathic symptoms often start gradually and then get worse. Deep proximal aching pain is the first sign in the affected limb. Burning pain in the cutaneous distribution of the affected nerve is frequent. Weakness and numbness usually appear over several hours to several days after the pain. The delay of the former symptoms is explained by the nerve infarction. On physical examination, most patients have pain and temperature sensory loss in the distribution of the affected nerve. A few patients have impairment of vibration and position sense. Hyporeflexia is also rare except in the ankles. In fact, tendon reflexes other than at the ankle are lost only if the femoral, musculocutaneous, or radial nerves are affected proximally [12, 18, 19]. The quantitative sensory testing (QST) is a tool to analyse the perception in response to external stimuli of controlled intensity. It has been used for the early diagnosis and follow-up of small fibre neuropathies. Although the QST is time-consuming and it is modified also in non-neuropathic pain as in rheumatoid arthritis and inflammatory myalgia, it cannot be taken alone as a conclusive demonstration of PN [20]. The QST is helpful to quantify the effects of treatments on allodynia and hyperalgesia and may reveal a differential efficacy of treatments on different pain components (grade A) [20]. According to EFNS international guidelines, to evaluate hyperalgesia in PN, it is recommended to use simple tools such as a brush and at least one high-intensity weighted pinprick or von Frey filament. The evaluation of pain in response to thermal stimuli is best performed by using the thermotest which is recommended for pathophysiological research or treatment trials. The DN4 may be a useful instrument for the daily diagnostic of PN in CTD [21].

5. Diagnosis and clinical results

In patient with multiorgan involvement and mononeuropathy multiplex, the diagnosis of vasculitic neuropathy is usually easy. However, the diagnosis may be more difficult in less typical presentations of CTD or when peripheral neuropathy is the unique manifestation of the disease. The diagnosis of peripheral neuropathy in CTD particularly in atypical situation is based first on clinical and physical examinations. Electromyography confirms even an underlying axonal neuropathy. The most characteristic electromyographic finding in vasculitic neuropathy described in the previous series is axonal degeneration with multifocal distribution. The typical feature is a low sensory nerve and compound muscle action potential amplitudes in a non-length-dependent distribution with normal or minimally reduced conduction velocities [15, 17, 22, 23]. A partial conduction block is rare, and it is seen transiently and early in stage of nerve ischemia [12]. Laboratory tests may be helpful in establishing the presence of systemic vasculitis or identifying previously undiagnosed connective tissue disease. Evaluation of patients with suspected neuropathy in CTD should include liver and kidney function tests, erythrocyte sedimentation rate, urinalysis as well as a complete blood count. The choice of immunological test including rheumatoid factor, antinuclear antibody, cryoglobulins, antineutrophil cytoplasmic autoantibody and serum complement depends on the clinical presentation of the patient. Nerve biopsy may be helpful in demonstrating vasculitic process. A concomitant muscle specimen is useful to increase diagnostic yield because of the patchy distribution of vasculitic lesions [18].

6. Particularity of PN in each CTD

6.1 Peripheral neuropathy in Sjögren syndrome

Sjögren syndrome is a CTD more prevalent in women at the age of menopause. It is characterized by sicca syndrome and other extra-glandular symptoms. Peripheral nervous involvement in Sjögren syndrome (SS) is reported with variable frequency because of diverse methods for detection of neuropathy and may precede the onset of the disease or be the initial diagnostic clue [24]. The most common feature is symmetrical distal sensory neuropathy, autonomic neuropathy and trigeminal sensory neuropathy. Mononeuritis multiplex, chronic inflammatory demyelinating neuropathy and motor neuropathy are less common [8].

6.1.1 Ganglionopathies

Sensory ganglionopathy is characterized by an impairment of kinesthetic awareness. Patients have the profound handicap of proprioceptive sense affecting larger joints. Electromyogram shows unelicitable sensory nerve action potentials, with preservation of compound motor action potentials [25]. When MRI is performed, it can reveal T2 hyperintensities limited to the gracile and cuneatus tracts of the dorsal spinal cord with sensory neuronopathies [26]. There are two mechanisms evoked in the pathogenesis of gangliopathies in SS. First, the cellular autoimmunity, confirmed by the infiltration of mononuclear and predominantly T cells in the dorsal root ganglia, is associated with cellular degeneration in the absence of vasculitis [25, 27, 28]. Second, recent studies have suggested that the presence of antibodies against the G-bodies, which are a subcellular aggregation of noncoding RNA intermediates and proteins, is associated to neuropathy [29, 30]. Moreover, It was reported that antineuronal antibodies were seen more frequently in Sjögren patients with severe peripheral neuropathy (PN) complications [25].

6.1.2 Small fibre neuropathies

Small fibre neuropathy is the most common PN manifestation of SS. It is a painful, sensory neuropathy affecting the nociceptive A-alpha and unmyelinated C-fibres. Small fibre neuropathy is reported with variable frequency. In the Hopkins Green Sjögren cohort, it was described as the most frequent manifestation [31]. The onset of small fibre neuropathy is usually subacute to chronic, occurring over weeks to months, although cases with hyperacute evolution of hours to days have been reported [27]. The cardinal clinical symptom of isolated small fibre neuropathy is an excruciating burning pain. The physical examination reveals a selective impairment in small-fibre modalities of pinprick and temperature, with relatively preserved vibratory sense and proprioception. The diagnosis of small fibre neuropathy is based on skin biopsy, which assesses the low density of intraepidermal nerve fibres [25, 32].

6.1.3 Sensorimotor polyneuropathies

The majority of studies reported that axonal polyneuropathies as the most frequent type of PN in SS. The onset of sensorimotor polyneuropathy is usually subacute or chronic. The axonal sensory neuropathies are characterized by proprioceptive sensory loss and motor reflexes, and there are diminished sensory nerve action potentials in electromyogram [25]. The sensory symptoms, however, are gradually accompanied by muscle weakness in a distal, symmetrical distribution [32].

6.1.4 Multiple mononeuropathy

It is the transduction of vasculitic neuropathy, and it is very uncommon in SS reported in 0–5% in previous studies. It is usually associated with extra-glandular manifestations [25, 27, 33–35]. Patients with SS and presenting mononeuritis multiplex should be assessed for cryoglobulinemia polyclonal (types II and III) rather than monoclonal (type I) mainly when there is high-titer rheumatoid factor positivity or when there is disproportionate C4 hypocomplementemia, with normal levels of C3. When nerve biopsy is performed, it may show a lymphocytic or necrotizing vasculitis [32].

6.1.5 Cranial neuropathies

The most common cranial neuropathy in SS is the trigeminal neuropathy, which is usually progressive and can be bilateral and requires symptomatic treatment. Motor dysfunction of cranial nerves is less common, and the facial nerve is the most cranial nerve targeted. The acute onset of cranial neuropathy is due to vasculitic mechanism especially when associated with equally rapid development of multiple mononeuropathies in the extremities [25].

6.1.6 Demyelinating neuropathies

Demyelinating neuropathy is a rare manifestation of SS [32, 33]. Cases of chronic idiopathic demyelinating polyneuropathy have been the subject of case reports in Sjögren patients but have not been substantially described in larger case series. The most common neurophysiologic finding in demyelinating neuropathies was demyelination of the motor nerves [36–38]. The onset of this neuropathy is subacute and characterized by severe proximal and distal weakness and proprioceptive sensory deficit. Treatment with steroid and sometimes with intravenous immune globulins may be effective [32, 39].

6.1.7 Autonomic neuropathy

Autonomic neuropathy is the rarest type of peripheral nerve involvement in SS because it is usually underdiagnosed. The clinical manifestations of autonomic neuropathy will vary depending on the organs which are affected. Symptoms range from urinary symptoms to severe disabling postural hypotension [27, 32, 38]. In recent studies, autonomic dysfunction is associated with the severity of fatigue in patients with primary SS. However, no association was detected between autonomic dysfunction and exocrine function in these patients [32, 40].

6.2 Peripheral neuropathy in systemic erythematosus lupus

Systemic lupus erythematosus is a multisystem autoimmune disorder with a broad spectrum of clinical presentations as cutaneous, renal and articular manifestations (**Figure 1**). Affected patients typically have subacute or chronic distal symmetrical polyneuropathies with predominant sensory symptoms. Distal symmetrical axonal degeneration is the major feature of most cases, although other types of peripheral neuropathy have been described [12, 41]. Oomatia reported the subtypes of peripheral neuropathy (PN) attributable to SLE in a group of 82 patients out of 2097 and detailed in **Table 2** [42]. Other features such as Guillain-Barré syndrome, plexopathy and autonomic neuropathy are very low in all series

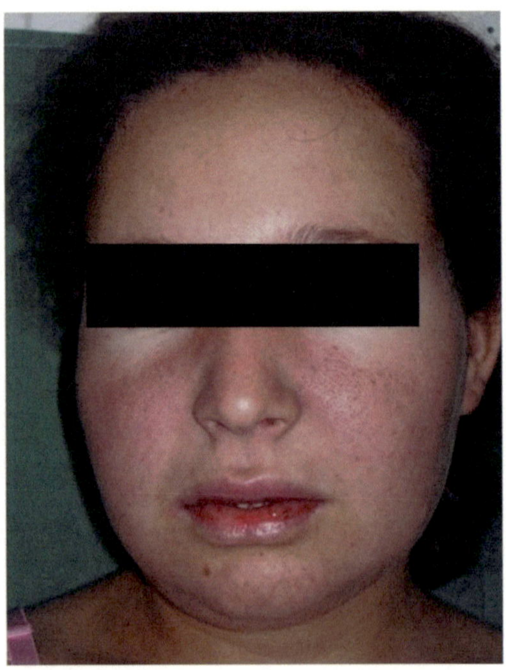

Figure 1.
Butterfly rash in systemic lupus erythematosus.

Type of peripheral neuropathy	Frequency no. (%)
Axonal neuropathies	46 (56.1)
Sensory axonal polyneuropathy	19 (23.2)
Sensorimotor axonal polyneuropathy	21 (25.6)
Mononeuritis multiplex	6 (7.3)
Small fibre neuropathies	14 (17.1)
Demyelinating polyneuropathies	
Acute inflammatory demyelinating polyneuropathy	1 (1.2)
Sensory demyelinating polyneuropathy	1 (1.2)
Mixed axonal-demyelinating sensorimotor polyneuropathy	3 (3.6)
Plexopathy	1 (1.2)

Table 2.
Type of peripheral neuropathy in SLE (adapted from peripheral neuropathies in systemic lupus erythematous/ Oomatia et al.) [42].

[41]. In recent data, small fibre neuropathy is more frequent in SLE, and the decreased intraepidermal nerve fibre density of unmyelinated fibres is a diagnostic test [42]. The mechanisms of peripheral neuropathy in SLE are unclear. Several factors have been reported particularly small-vessel vasculitis and lesions induced by autoimmune antibodies and immune complexes. In series, where nerve biopsy is performed, the anatomopathologic aspect was perivascular mononuclear cell infiltration and variable intimal thickening without necrotizing vasculitis. The presence of necrotizing vasculitis is possible and constitutes a prognostic factor of the disease [12, 41, 43]. Endoneurial mononuclear cell infiltration and increased class II antigen expression were also noticed [12, 43].

6.3 Peripheral neuropathy in systemic sclerosis

Systemic sclerosis is a rare connective tissue disease with a prevalence of 1 in 10,000 [44]. It is characterized by symmetrical, widespread thickening of the skin (**Figure 2**) [45]. The prevalence of peripheral neuropathy is unknown with reported ranges in retrospective studies varying from 0.01 to 14% of patients [46, 47]. Vascular-dependent neuropathy is the principal mechanism inducing a distal symmetric, mainly sensory polyneuropathy as in other connective tissue diseases [13, 46, 47]. Cranial mononeuropathies can also occur, mainly the trigeminal nerve, leading to numbness and dysesthesias in the face. Rarely the seventh and ninth cranial neuropathies are affected [11]. The electrophysiological features are those of sensory axonopathy [11]. Rare cases of mononeuritis multiplex have been mentioned in the course of limited SSc (CREST: calcinosis, Raynaud's phenomenon, oesophageal dysmotility, sclerodactyly, telangiectasia) and are due to a necrotizing vasculitis [11].

6.4 Peripheral neuropathy in mixed connective tissue disease

Mixed connective tissue disease is defined as the overlap of SLE, SSc and PM, with a high titer of extractable nuclear antigen and its ribonucleoprotein component [48]. Mild distal axonal polyneuropathy was exceptionally reported in 2 of 20 patients with mixed connective tissue disease, but there has not been a detailed study of the neuropathy or its treatment [48].

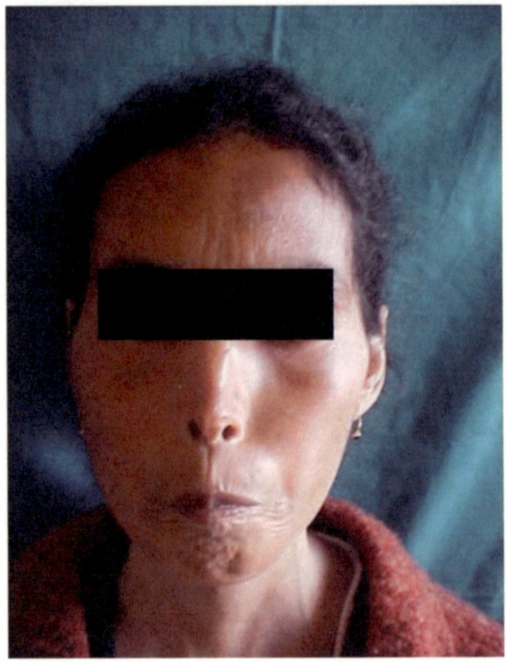

Figure 2.
Sclerosis of the face in systemic sclerosis.

6.5 Peripheral neuropathy in dermatomyositis and polymyositis

Nerve involvement in patients with DM is mediated through membrane attack complex (MAC) formation, leading to nerve injury. This entity called "neuromyositis" was first reported in 1890 [49]. Further studies showed a frequency of 7.5% in DM or PM patients with polyneuropathy [50]. Neuropathy due to DM is difficult to diagnose due to necessity of excluding other comorbid etiologic conditions and heterogeneity of muscular manifestations [49]. Nerve biopsy may reveal endothelial vascular injury, and immunohistochemical stains revealed increased expression of perivascular VEGF and demyelinization associated or not with inflammation [51].

7. Treatment of peripheral neuropathy in CTD

7.1 General approach

There are no treatment guidelines specific to each CTD. In general, the management of PN is based on symptomatic treatment of pain as in other causes of neuropathies. Typically, patients with painful polyneuropathies respond to drugs known to be effective for neuropathic pain, including tricyclic antidepressants and a variety of antiepileptic drugs as gabapentin and pregabalin, which is preferred because of its better bioavailability [52]. Concerning the antidepressants, international guidelines provide the same level of recommendation for nonselective tricyclic antidepressants and serotonin-norepinephrine reuptake inhibitors (SNRIs). Most clinical trials showed that the efficacy of SNRIs is lower than that of tricyclic antidepressants. However, tricyclic antidepressants have more side effects in elderly and are contraindicated in patients with glaucoma, prostate hypertrophy or some cardiac conduction disturbances. Venlafaxine is a SNRI who has shown efficacy in painful polyneuropathies of different origins [53]. In CTD, PN is mainly due to vasculitic and immune abnormalities. So when vasculitic neuropathy is diagnosed, corticosteroids should be promptly introduced to recover sensory and motor deficits [3]. Most authors recommend starting oral prednisone at high dose of 1 mg/kg per day. In severe cases, intravenous pulses of methylprednisolone of one 1 g for 3–5 days might be appropriate for initial treatment. This treatment should be maintained during the subacute phase, and after 6 to 8 weeks, the treatment should be tapered progressively. Immunosuppressant therapy is associated to corticosteroids in severe forms of vasculitic neuropathy or in systemic vasculitic PN. Cyclophosphamide seems to be the most effective drug for induction of remission and improvement of survival in non-viral systemic vasculitides [18]. Most patients need 3–12 months of cyclophosphamide induction therapy before they can be switched to a maintenance immunosuppressant [54]. Immunosuppressant used as a maintenance therapy is azathioprine, methotrexate and mycophenolate mofetil [55]. Intravenous immunoglobulin is a safe treatment used in serious systemic PN with clinical benefit [18].

7.2 Particularities of treatment in each CTD

Therapeutic strategies of small fibre neuropathy in SS are still unclear. Carbamazepine is generally the first-line agent for trigeminal neuralgia. The use

PNS manifestation	First-line treatment approach	Treatment of refractory cases
Polyneuropathy	Neurotrophic agents (tricyclic antidepressants, SNRI (duloxetine, venlafaxine), anticonvulsants (gabapentin, pregabalin)) (glucocorticoids (1 mg/kg/day of prednisone equivalent)) Severe forms: immunosuppressants (azathioprine, mycophenolate mofetil, cyclophosphamide)	Carbamazepine High-dose IVIG PEX Rituximab
Mononeuropathy single/ multiple	Systemic glucocorticoids (1–2 mg/kg/ day of prednisone equivalent or pulses of methylprednisolone 500/1000 mg for 3–5 days with long-term dosage reduction) IV Cyclophosphamide	Rituximab, IVIG, PEX Mycophenolate mofetil Azathioprine
Small fibre neuropathy	Neurotrophic agents (tricyclic antidepressants, SNRI (duloxetine, venlafaxine), anticonvulsants (gabapentin, pregabalin)), topical anaesthetics Analgesics	Immunosuppressants IVIG Psychological support
Acute inflammatory demyelinating polyradiculoneuropathy (GBS)	High-dose IVIG PEX Cardiorespiratory supporting measures	Glucocorticoids (1 mg/ kg/day of prednisone 1000 mg for 3 days) Equivalent or pulses of methylprednisolone and immunosuppressants – cyclophosphamide
Cranial neuropathy	Glucocorticoids (1 mg/kg/day of prednisone equivalent) with long-term dosage reduction Spontaneous recovery possible for oculomotor involvement	Cyclophosphamide immunosuppressants as maintenance treatment

PNS: peripheral nervous system; SNRI: serotonin-norepinephrine reuptake inhibitors; IVIG: intravenous immunoglobulins; PEX: plasma exchange; GBS: Guillain Barré Syndrom.

Table 3.
Treatment options available for peripheral nervous system involvement in patients with SLE (adapted from PNS involvement in SLE/A. Bortoluzzi et al.) [60].

of other antiepileptic agents such as gabapentin should be prescribed with slow titration to minimize its side effects particularly over somnolence and fatigue. The duration of therapeutic trial should be at least 3 months. The secondary amine tricyclic antidepressants such as nortriptyline and desipramine have fewer anticholinergic side effects and a proven efficacy in neuropathic pain, and so they may be slowly prescribed in patients with SS. The use of new immunosuppressant agents mainly monoclonal antibody directed against CD20 antigen on B cells as rituximab and the tumour necrosis factor (TNF)-alpha inhibitors such as adalimumab has been reported to be efficient in the small fibre neuropathies occurring in SS [25]. The management of axonal polyneuropathy is based on a symptomatic treatment; corticosteroids and immunosuppressors are discussed in the case of motor neuropathy with rapid progression [25]. In the case of multiple mononeuropathy, the presence of vasculitis is associated with a good response to immunosuppressive therapy [34]. There is evidence supporting the use of immunoglobulin therapy in Sjögren-associated sensorimotor and non-ataxic sensory neuropathy from retrospective and observational cohorts and case reports [56, 57].

In SLE, there are no clear guidelines on the treatment of peripheral neuropathy. Induction treatments with glucocorticoids with or without immunosuppressant agents are indicated in the situation of active vasculitic neuropathy [58]. In the case of necrotizing vasculitis, treatment with plasmapheresis, steroids and immunosuppressant has led to improvement [59, 60]. The definitions of response to treatment are variable between studies. Overall, the rate of global response (complete or partial) is more than 50% [41] (**Table 3**).

In SSc, there is not enough data regarding the response of scleroderma-associated neuropathy to immunosuppression [11, 61]. However, this therapy seems to be effective in mononeuritis multiplex and sensorimotor polyneuropathy with inflammatory process [11]. In DM/PM the treatment of PN is based on corticosteroids and immunosuppressant agents depending on the severity of the clinic presentation [51].

PNS, peripheral nervous system; SNRI, serotonin-norepinephrine reuptake inhibitors; IVIG, intravenous immunoglobulins; PEX, plasma exchange; GBS, Guillain-Barré syndrome.

8. Conclusion

8.1 Final considerations

PN is one of the possible neurologic manifestations encountered by physicians in CTD. Coexistence of both conditions is explained by immune-mediated factors particularly a vasculitis of peripheral nerve. Therefore, it is important to take a detailed medical history and examination and then adequate investigations to assess for an underlying systemic autoimmune diseases that may be associated with the neuropathy. Pure sensory and sensorimotor neuropathies are the most common PN features in these disorders. Acute to subacutely evolving multifocal or asymmetric neuropathy suggests a vasculitic cause. This situation constitutes a prognostic factor of the disease and requires prompt treatment with steroids and immunosuppressant agents. The treatment of PN in CTD progresses in three fronts: first, to identify the type of PN through the medical history and physical exam; second, to precise the pathogenic mechanism of neuropathy via clinical presentation, electromyographic data and in unclear situation the nerve biopsy and finally, the efficient control of pain. Corticosteroids remain the mainstay of treatment for vasculitic neuropathy in CTD.

8.2 Futures directions

Although much is known about the PN in CTD, particularly its pathogenesis and its clinical aspects, further experience needs to be gained especially in the treatment with prospective trials to identify indications and precise efficacy for cytotoxic agents, intravenous immunoglobulin, plasma exchange and new biological drugs. In future, we need also further studies to precise clear guidelines to diagnose PN related to CTD such as more specific features in the electromyogram and neuromuscular biopsy. Moreover, in the treatment approach of PN in CTD, we need further researches to identify curative drugs targeting the pathogenesis pathways rather than the symptomatic and the previous conventional therapy.

Conflict of interest

There is no conflict of interest.

Author details

Mouna Snoussi*, Faten Frikha and Zouhir Bahloul
Department of Internal Medicine, Medical School of Sfax, Tunisia

*Address all correspondence to: mounasnoussi23@yahoo.fr

References

[1] Kumar TS, Aggarwal A. Approach to a patient with connective tissue disease. Indian Journal of Pediatrics. 2010;**77**:1157-1164. DOI: 10.1007/s12098-010-0207

[2] Servioli L, Pérez C, Consani S, et al. Prevalence and characteristics of immuno-mediated neuropathies in a group of patients with autoimmune diseases. Journal of Clinical Neuromuscular Disease. 2007;**9**:285-290

[3] Matthew NM, Morgenlander JC. Peripheral neuropathy and connective tissue disease. Postgraduate Medicine. 1997;**102**(5):65-75. DOI: 10.3810/pgm.1997.11.367

[4] Matthew Grantz MD. Unusual peripheral neuropathies. Part II: Intrinsic reactive causes. Seminars in Neurology. 2010;**30**:396-404

[5] Ilniczky S, Kamondi A, Arányi Z, et al. Simultaneous central and peripheral nervous system involvement in systemic lupus erythematosus. Ideggyógyászati Szemle. 2007;**60**:398-402

[6] Omdal R, Mellgren SI, Goransson L, et al. Small nerve fiber involvement in systemic lupus erythematosus: A controlled study. Arthritis and Rheumatism. 2002;**46**:1228-1232. DOI: 10.1002/art.10303

[7] Norman L. Peripheral Neuropathy: When the Numbness, Weakness, and Pain Won't Stop. New York: American Academy of Neurology Press Demos Medical; 2007

[8] Cojocaru IM, Cojocaru M, Silosi I, Vrabie CD. Peripheral nervous system in autoimmune diseases. MAEDICA – A Journal of Clinical Medicine. 2014;**9**(3):289-294

[9] Mendell JR, Sahenk Z. Clinical practice. Painful sensory neuropathy. The New England Journal of Medicine. 2003;**348**(13):1243-1255. DOI: 10.1056/NEJMcp022282

[10] Rosenbaum R. Neuromuscular complications of connective tissue diseases. Muscle & Nerve. 2001;**24**:154-169

[11] Poncelet AN, Connolly MK. Peripheral neuropathy in scleroderma. Muscle & Nerve. 2003;**28**(3):330-335. DOI:10.1002/mus.10439

[12] Richard K, Olney MD. Neuropathies associated with connective tissue disease. Seminars in Neurology. 1998;**18**(1):63-72. DOI: 10.1055/s-2008-1040862

[13] Spirin NN, Bulanova VA, Pizova NV, Shilkina NP. Peripheral nervous system lesion syndromes in connective tissue diseases. Neuroscience and Behavioral Physiology. 2007;**37**(1):1-6. DOI: 10.1007/s11055-007-0141-1

[14] Dyck PJ, Conn DL, Okazaki H. Necrotizing angiopathic neuropathy. Mayo Clinic Proceedings. 1972;**47**:461-475

[15] Ropert A, Metral S. Conduction block in neuropathies with necrotizing vasculitis. Muscle & Nerve. 1990;**13**:102-105. DOI: 10.1002/mus.880130203

[16] Chalk CH, Conn DL, Dyck PJ. Vasculitic neuropathy. In: Dyck PJ, Thomas PK, Griffin JW, Low PA, Poduslo JF, editors. Peripheral Neuropathy. Vol. 2. Philadelphia: WB Saunders Co; 1992. pp. 1424-1430

[17] Kissel JT, Mendell JR. Vasculitic neuropathy. In: Dyck PJ, ed. Peripheral neuropathy: New concepts and treatments. Neurologic Clinics. 1992;**10**(3):761-781

[18] Gwathmey KG, Burns TM, Collins MP, Dyck PJB. Vasculitic neuropathies. Lancet Neurology. 2014;**13**:67-82

[19] Hellmann DB, Laing TJ, Petri M, Whiting-O'Keefe Q Parry GJ. Mononeuritis multiplex: The yield of evaluations for occult rheumatic diseases. Medicine (Baltimore). 1988;**67**:145-153

[20] Cruccua G, Sommera C, Anandd P, Attala N, Baronf R, Garcia-Larreaa L, et al. EFNS guidelines on neuropathic pain assessment: Revised 2009. European Journal of Neurology. 2010;**17**:1010-1018. DOI: 10.1111/j.1468-1331.2010.02969.x

[21] Bouhassiraa D, Attala N, Alchaarb H, Boureauc F, Brochetd B, Bruxellee J, et al. Comparison of pain syndromes associated with nervous or somatic lesions and development of a new neuropathic pain diagnostic questionnaire (DN4). Pain. 2005;**114**:29-36

[22] Bouche P, Leger JM, Travers MA, Cathala HP, Castaigne P. Peripheral neuropathy in systemic vasculitis: Clinical and electrophysiologic study-of 22 patients. Neurology. 1986;**36**:1598-1602

[23] Parry GJ, Brown MJ. Selective fiber vulnerability in acute ischemic neuropathy. Annals of Neurology. 1982;**11**:147-154. DOI: 10.1002/ana.410110207

[24] Perzyńska-Mazan J, Maślińska M, Gasik R. Neurological manifestations of primary Sjögren's syndrome. Reumatologia. 2018;**56**(2):99-105

[25] Birnbaum J. Peripheral nervous system manifestations of Sjögren syndrome: Clinical patterns, diagnostic paradigms, etiopathogenesis, and therapeutic strategies. The Neurologist. 2010;**16**:287-297. DOI: 10.1097/NRL.0b013e3181ebe59f

[26] Mori K, Koike H, Misu K, et al. Spinal cord magnetic resonance imaging demonstrates sensory neuronal involvement and clinical severity in neuronopathy associated with Sjogren's syndrome. Journal of Neurology, Neurosurgery, and Psychiatry. 2001;**71**:488-492

[27] Mori K, Iijima M, Koike H, et al. The wide spectrum of clinical manifestations in Sjogren's syndrome-associated neuropathy. Brain. 2005;**128**:2518-2534. DOI: 10.1093/brain/awh605

[28] Griffin JW, Cornblath DR, Alexander E, et al. Ataxic sensory neuropathy and dorsal root ganglionitis associated with Sjogren's syndrome. Annals of Neurology. 1990;**27**:304-315. DOI: 10.1002/ana.410270313

[29] Bhanji RA, Eystathioy T, Chan EK, et al. Clinical and serological features of patients with autoantibodies to GW/P bodies. Clinical Immunology. 2007;**125**:247-256. DOI: 10.1016/j.clim.2007.07.016

[30] Malinow K, Yannakakis GD, Glusman SM, et al. Subacute sensory neuronopathy secondary to dorsal root ganglionitis in primary Sjogren's syndrome. Annals of Neurology. 1986;**20**:535-537. DOI: 10.1002/ana.410200416

[31] Birnbaum J. Peripheral neuropathy is an uncommon cause of neuropathic symptoms in Sjogren's patients. Arthritis and Rheumatism. 2009;**60**(suppl 10):506

[32] Pavlakis PP, Alexopoulos H, Kosmidis ML, Mamali I, Moutsopoulos HM, Tzioufas AG, et al. Peripheral neuropathies in Sjögren's syndrome: A critical update on clinical features and pathogenetic mechanisms. Journal of Autoimmunity. 2012;**39**:27-33. DOI: 10.1016/j.jaut.2012.01.003

[33] Grant IA, Hunder GG, Homburger HA, et al. Peripheral neuropathy

associated with sicca complex. Neurology. 1997;**48**:855-862

[34] Terrier B, Lacroix C, Guillevin L, et al. Diagnostic and prognostic relevance of neuromuscular biopsy in primary Sjogren's syndrome-related neuropathy. Arthritis and Rheumatism. 2007;**57**:1520-1529. DOI: 10.1002/art.23102

[35] Delalande S, de Seze J, Fauchais AL, et al. Neurologic manifestations in primary Sjogren syndrome: A study of 82 patients. Medicine (Baltimore). 2004;**83**:280-291

[36] Novak V, Freimer ML, Kissel JT, et al. Autonomic impairment in painful neuropathy. Neurology. 2001;**56**:861-868

[37] Rigamonti A, Lauria G, Balgera R, et al. Subacute inflammatory polyradiculopathy polyradiculopathy associated with Sjogren's syndrome. Muscle & Nerve. 2009;**39**:855-857. DOI: 10.1002/mus.21274

[38] Pou Serradell A, Vinas Gaya J. 3 cases of rare peripheral neuropathies associated with primary Gougerot-Sjogren syndrome. Revue Neurologique (Paris). 1993;**149**:481-484

[39] Dalakas MC. Advances in the diagnosis, pathogenesis and treatment of CIDP. Nature Reviews. Neurology. 2011. DOI: 10.1038/nrneurol.2011.121

[40] Mandl T, Hammar O, Theander E, Wollmer P, Ohlsson B. Autonomic nervous dysfunction development in patients with primary Sjogren's syndrome: A follow-up study. Rheumatology (Oxford, England). 2010;**49**:1101e6. DOI: 10.1093/rheumatology/keq042

[41] Toledano P, Orueta R, Rodríguez-Pintó I, Valls-Solé J, Cervera R, Espinosa G. Peripheral nervous system involvement in systemic lupus erythematosus: Prevalence, clinical and immunological characteristics, treatment and outcome of a large cohort from a single Centre. Autoimmunity Reviews. 2017 Jul;**16**(7):750-755. DOI: 10.1016/j.autrev.2017.05.011

[42] Oomatia A, Fang H, Petri M, Birnbaum J. Peripheral neuropathies in systemic lupus erythematosus. Arthritis & Rheumatology. April 2014;**66**(4):1000-1009. DOI: 10.1002/art.38302

[43] McCombe PA, McLeod JG, Pollard JD, Guo Y-P, Ingall TJ. Peripheral sensorimotor and autonomic neuropathy associated with systemic lupus erythematosus. Brain. 1987;**110**:S33-S549

[44] LeRoy EC, Silver RM. Systemic sclerosis and related syndromes: Epidemiology, pathology, and pathogenesis. In: Schumacher HR, Klippel JH, Koopman WJ, editors. Primer on the Rheumatic Diseases. 10th ed. Vol. 1993. Atlanta: Arthritis Foundation. pp. 118-120

[45] Medsger TA, Steen V. Systemic sclerosis and related syndromes: Clinical features and treatment. In: Schumacher HR, Klippel JH, Koopman WJ, editors. Primer on the Rheumatic Diseases. 10th ed. Atlanta: Arthritis Foundation; 1993. pp. 120-127

[46] Tagliafico A, Panico N, Resmini E, Derchi LE, Ghio M, Martinoli C. The role of ultrasound imaging in the evaluation of peripheral nerve in systemic sclerosis (scleroderma). European Journal of Radiology. 2011;**77**(3):377-382. DOI: 10.1016/j.ejrad.2009.08.010

[47] Frech TM, Smith G, Reily M, Chamberlain J, Murtaugh MA, Penrod J, et al. Peripheral neuropathy: A complication of systemic sclerosis. Clinical Rheumatology. 2013;**32**:885-888. DOI: 10.1007/s10067-013-2206-6

[48] Bennett RM, Bong DM, Spargo BH. Neuropsychiatric problems in mixed tissue disease. The American Journal of Medicine. 1978;**65**:955-962

[49] Nguyen TP, Bangert C, Biliciler S, Athar P, Sheikh K. Dermatomyositis-associated sensory neuropathy: A unifying pathogenic hypothesis. Journal of Clinical Neuromuscular Disease. 2014;**16**:7-11. DOI: 10.1097/CND.0000000000000048

[50] Wang Y, Cui LY, Chen L, et al. Nerve conduction studies in patients with dermatomyositis or polymyositis. Chinese Medical Journal. 2010;**123**:523-526

[51] Onder H, GökcemYıldız F, Temucin ÇM. Neuromyositis: Clinical and electrophysiological study of 8 cases. Journal of Medicine and Medical Science. 2015;**4**(7):347-350

[52] Cruccu G, Truini A. A review of neuropathic pain: From guidelines to clinical practice. Pain and Therapy. 2017;**6**(Suppl 1):S35-S42

[53] Chetty S, Baalbergen E, Bhigjee AI, Kamerman P, Ouma J, Raath R, et al. Clinical practice guidelines for management of neuropathic. South African Medical Journal. 2012;**102**(5):312-325

[54] Langford CA. Vasculitis. The Journal of Allergy and Clinical Immunology. 2003;**111**:S602-S612

[55] Langford CA. How can relapses be detected and prevented in primary systemic small-vessel vasculitides? Best Practice & Research. Clinical Rheumatology. 2005;**19**:307-320. DOI: 10.1016/j.berh.2004.11.003

[56] Rist S, Sellam J, Hachulla E, et al. Experience of intravenous immunoglobulin therapy in neuropathy associated with primary Sjogren's syndrome: A national multicentric retrospective study. Arthritis Care and Research. 2011;**63**:133944

[57] Morozumi S, Kawagashira Y, Iijima M, et al. Intravenous immunoglobulin treatment for painful sensory neuropathy associated with Sjogren's syndrome. Journal of the Neurological Sciences. 2009;**279**:5761

[58] Govoni M, Bortoluzzi A, Padovan M, Silvagni E, Borrelli M, Donelli F, et al. The diagnosis and clinical management of the neuropsychiatric manifestations of lupus. Journal of Autoimmunity. 2016;**74**:41-72. DOI: 10.1016/j.jaut.2016.06.013

[59] Florica B, Aghdassi E, Su J, Gladman DD, Urowitz MB, Fortin PR. Peripheral neuropathy in patients with systemic lupus erythematosus. Seminars in Arthritis and Rheumatism. 2011;**41**:203-211. DOI: 10.1016/j.semarthrit.2011.04.001

[60] Bortoluzzi A, Silvagni E, Furini F, Piga M, Govoni M. Peripheral nervous system involvement in systemic lupus erythematosus: A review of the evidence. Clinical and Experimental Rheumatology. 2018. [Epub ahead of print]

[61] Amarala TN, Peres FA, Lapa AT, Marques-Neto JF, Appenzeller S. Neurologic involvement in scleroderma: A systematic review. Seminars in Arthritis and Rheumatism. 2013;**43**:335-347. DOI: 10.1016/j.semarthrit.2013.05.002

Chapter 4

Working Hand Syndrome: A New Definition of Nonclassified Polyneuropathy Condition

Gökhan Özdemir

Abstract

The aim of this chapter was to define an unexplained nonclassified polyneuropathy condition as a new neurological disease. This new diagnosis of occupation-related polyneuropathy has been named as "working hand syndrome (WHS)." This study collected and compared clinical and electrophysiological analyses data from healthy controls, WHS patients, carpal tunnel syndrome (CTS) patients, and polyneuropathy patients. The WHS patients presented to the clinic with pain, numbness, tingling, and burning sensations in their hands that increased significantly during rest and nighttime. However, there was no weakness in the muscles, and the deep tendon reflexes were normal in this disease. The patients had all been working in physically demanding jobs requiring the use of their hands/arms for at least 1 year, but no vibrating tools were used by the patients. All of the cases were men. I suppose that overload caused by an action repeated chronically by the hand/arm may impair the sensory nerves in mentioned hand/arm. In patients with these complaints, for a definitive diagnosis, similar diseases must be excluded. Nonetheless, the specific electrophysiological finding that the sural nerves are normal on the lower sides, as well as the occurrence of sensory axonal polyneuropathy in the sensory nerves without a significant effect on velocity and latency in the work-ups of the upper extremity are enough to make a diagnosis.

Keywords: working hand syndrome (WHS)

1. Inclusion

Polyneuropathies (PNP) are disorders of the peripheral nervous system that indicates any disorder of the peripheral nervous system. Polyneuropathy is one of the most prevalent neurologic conditions. Polyneuropathy has an estimated prevalence of 5–8% in the general population. However, if there are one or more risk factors involved, this rate can increase to 12–17%. Various systemic diseases, exposure to toxicity, drugs, infections, and hereditary diseases are considered causes. Young patients are much more likely to have a polyneuropathy on a genetic basis, elderly patients are much more likely to have idiopathic polyneuropathy, and middle-age patients are more likely to have acquired polyneuropathy. It needs to be done that family history and other important details of the individual's history and examination. Family history should focus on illnesses associated with neuropathy, such as diabetes mellitus, hypothyroidism, renal failure, hepatic disorder, human immunodeficiency virus infection, and dysproteinemic disorders (10% of peripheral neuropathies are associated with dysproteinemias) and in those receiving chemotherapy and cancer. In the developed world, the most common cause of peripheral neuropathy is diabetes mellitus. Patients with cancer may develop neuropathy depending to nutritional deficiency and chemotherapy side effects. But the etiology of 20–25% of these neuropathies remains uncertain [1–3].

The clinical manifestations of peripheral neuropathy vary widely that weakness, fatigue, hypesthesia, ataxia, autonomic symptoms, and positive symptoms include cramps, twitching, and myokymia. Sensorimotor peripheral neuropathies are the most common form of neuropathy. Usually, there is a progression from distal to proximal. Diminished deep tendon reflexes, distal muscle weakness, and atrophy are common in advanced cases. Most neuropathies are chronic and progressive. Peripheral neuropathy may be symmetrically generalized, multifocal, or focal. Most neuropathies are symmetric and length-dependent. Chronic symmetrical polyneuropathy is the most common type of polyneuropathy and usually evolves over months. Sensory or motor symptoms in a more diffuse, involving both proximal and distal limbs in length-independent pattern. In these cases reflexes are globally reduced or absent. The earliest symptoms of polyneuropathy are usually sensory abnormalities. Sensory symptoms start in the feet, which are supplied by the longest axons. Pathologic mechanisms in peripheral neuropathy are distal axonopathy, myelinopathy, and neuronopathy. The symptoms ascend insidiously up the leg. The upper limb involvement may never occur. Development of symptoms in the hands and feet at the same time is atypical for a length-dependent neuropathy and may indicate coexisting disorder [2, 3].

One of the most common causes of neuropathic pain in the hands is physical compression of the nerves, known as compression neuropathy. Carpal tunnel syndrome (CTS) and cubital tunnel syndrome are examples. Direct injury to a nerve, interruption of its blood supply, or inflammation may also cause neuropathic pain.

Anamnesis, neurological checkup, and electrophysiological work-up are recommended for diagnosis [1–3].

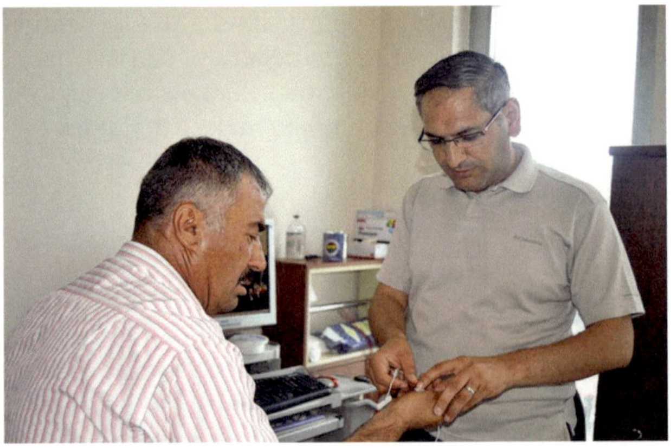

2. Working hand syndrome

Working hand syndrome patients have neuropathic pain in their hands, and axonal neuropathy is detected only in the sensorial neurons of the upper extremity. The common trait for these patients is the fact that they used their hands/arms during heavy labor. I think that a significant number of patients as this should not to be underestimated in the general population. Common traits among the patients include man sex, use of the arms and hands in heavy labor, neuropathic pain in their hands, and axonal polyneuropathy in the sensory median and ulnar nerves. The average age of the patients is 45.7 ± 20.4 years in working hand syndrome (WHS).

None of the WHS cases have systemic disease, and all of the cases are men. The use of the upper extremity while working a physically demanding job (construction worker, farmer, forester, crushing, tire repairer) requiring the use of the hands/arms for at least 1 year; presentation with pain, numbness, tingling and burning sensations (neuropathic) in the hands and fingers that increases significantly during rest and nighttime in the WHS [1].

3. Etiopathogenesis

Pathology in the sensory nerves can cause neuropathic pain. Sensory polyneuropathy is one of the most common causes of neuropathic pain. It is believed that WHS is likely a sensory neuropathy with such a mechanism as axonal polyneuropathy, because the ulnar nerve is more affected than the median nerve in the upper extremities in polyneuropathies. I posit that an overload caused by an action repeated chronically by the hand/arm may impair the sensory nerves in the said hand/arm. Not only the peripheral nervous system but also the local vessels may be affected. This process may result in vasoconstriction of the local vessels. This situation leads to hypoxia and a lack of nutrition in the sensory nerves. However, there is not a clear relation between WHS and its pathology. However, in my opinion, genetics, ergonomics, emotional stress, and biodynamic status play an important role in WHS, because this disease does not occur in everyone who is doing the same job [1].

4. Diagnosis

WHS is a polyneuropathy and occupational disease. Patients with WHS present with pain, numbness, tingling, and burning sensations in their hands that increases significantly during rest and nighttime. They also use their arms/hands for jobs that require heavy labor. The neurological examinations of patients with WHS are normal. Only the sensory nerves in the upper extremities are affected.

	Carpal tunnel syndrome	Hand-arm vibration syndrome	Chronic ıdiopathic axonal polyneuropathy	Working hand syndrome
Sural nerve	Normal	Normal	Decreased SNAP	Normal
The sensory median nerve distal latency/velocity	Delayed/Decreases	Delayed/Decreases	Normal/Normal	Normal/Normal
SNAP of the sensory median nerve	May be reduced	May be reduced	Reduced	Reduced
The sensory ulnar nerve distal latency/velocity	Normal/Normal	Delayed/Decreases	Normal/Normal	Normal/Normal
SNAP of the sensory ulnar nerve	Normal	May be reduced	Reduced	Reduced
CMAP of lower extremity motor nerves	Normal	Normal	Reduced	Normal

	Carpal tunnel syndrome	Hand-arm vibration syndrome	Chronic ıdiopathic axonal polyneuropathy	Working hand syndrome
The motor median nerve distal latency/velocity	May be delayed/ decreases	May be delayed/ decreases	Normal/Normal	Normal/Normal
CMAP of the motor median nerve	May be reduced	May be reduced	May be reduced	Normal
The motor ulnar nerve distal latency/velocity	Normal/Normal	Delayed/Decreases	Normal/Normal	Normal/Normal
CMAP of the motor ulnar nerve	Normal	May be reduced	May be reduced	Normal

SNAP, sensory nerve action potential; CMAP, compound muscle action potential.

Table 1.
Electrophysiological findings of working hand syndrome and similar diseases.

	Carpal tunnel syndrome	Hand-arm vibration syndrome	Chronic ıdiopathic axonal polyneuropathy	Working hand syndrome
Age	Intermediate and advanced ages	Young or middle ages	Intermediate and advanced ages	Young, middle or advanced ages
Gender	Female are generally affected	No significant gender differences	No significant gender differences	All male
Complaint	Neuropathic pain is often in the hands	Neuropathic pain is often in the hands	Especially neuropathic pain in the feet	Neuropathic pain is the hands
Risk factors	For example, rheumatism, pregnancy, diabetes, etc.	Continuous use of vibrating hand-held machinery	For example, diabetes, various cardiovascular risk factors, the metabolic syndrome, etc.	Patients used their hands/arms in heavy labor (no use of vibrating hand-held machinery)
Raynaud's phenomenon	No	Yes	No	No
Affected tissues	Only the median nerve	Median and ulnar nerves (motor and sensory nerves), blood vessels, nerves, muscles, and joints	Especially sural nerve and other sensory and motor nerves	Only the median and ulnar sensory nerves
Deep tendon reflexes	Unaffected	Usually unaffected	Usually decreases	Unaffected
Muscle weakness and atrophy	Advanced cases	Advanced cases	Advanced cases	No

Table 2.
Differential diagnosis of working hand syndrome.

For a definitive diagnosis:

1. All have been working in physically demanding jobs requiring the use of the hands/arms.

2. Patients exhibit neuropathic pain in their hands.

3. The exclusion of similar diseases (**Tables 1** and **2**).

4. Specific electrophysiological findings that the sural nerves are normal, as well as the occurrence of sensory axonal polyneuropathy in the sensory nerves without being greatly affected by speed and latency in the work-ups of the upper extremity, are enough to make a diagnosis [1].

5. Nerve conduction studies

The electromyographer plays an important role in the evaluation of patients with polyneuropathy. The results of nerve conduction studies and electromyography are useful in analyzing the underlying pathophysiology. The recording and measurement of the terminal latency, amplitude, duration of the evoked potential, and the conduction velocity. Nerve conduction studies are also valuable in differentiating whether a demyelinating process is acquired or inherited. Nerve conduction studies can identify the predominant pathophysiology (axonal loss or segmental demyelination) and establish whether sensory or motor findings predominate. In addition, the studies provide quantitating the severity and the distribution of the neuropathy. Electrophysiological work-ups show axonal damage (axonal neuropathy), demyelination (demyelinating neuropathy), and both (mix neuropathy). In the electrophysiological work-ups that involve distal latency, the amplitude, shape, and velocity of the motor and sensory nerves are checked. Axonal degeneration causes a decrease in amplitude, while demyelinating polyneuropathy causes delays in distal latencies and decreases in velocity. Acute axonal damage in the motor nerves can cause spontaneous activities in muscle fibers when checked with electromyography, where dilution in voluntary activity and chronic neurogenic motor unit potentials (MUP) are seen [1, 4].

The electrophysiological work-ups in the WHS are completed with standardized supramaximal percutaneous stimulation techniques. In the upper sides, a sensorial check-up is completed of the median and ulnar nerves. The sural nerves are used for a lower extremity sensory evaluation. For the median motor nerve evaluation, a 6–7 cm proximal of the abductor pollicis brevis muscle is supramaximally stimulated; the ulnar motor nerve is recorded from the abductor minimi muscle; the median sensorial nerve is recorded from the second finger; and the ulnar sensorial nerve is recorded from the fifth finger. For the sural nerves, the active electrode was placed between the lateral malleolus and the heel, and the reference electrode was placed 30 mm distally at the lateral edge of the foot. Supramaximal stimuli are applied at 13 cm proximal to the active electrode, just lateral to the midline of the calf. Amplitudes below 16 uV for the sensorial nerves in the upper sides and amplitudes below 10 uV for the sensorial nerves in the lower sensory sides (sural nerves) are considered the limits of sensory axonal neuropathy to assess its sensitivity and specificity. The use of an infrared lamp ensured that the temperature of the extremities during measurement has been done at 34°C or higher. In the electrophysiological findings of the WHS according to the normal, the distal latency and velocity of the median and ulnar sensorial nerves are similar in both hands. However, both the median sensory and ulnar sensory nerve amplitudes are decreased ($P < 0.05$). The motor nerve conduction work-ups of the upper and lower sides are similar in all differential diagnosis. The sural nerve results are similar on the lower sides in the normal, CTS, and WHS. The sural nerve results are significantly affected in the polyneuropathy ($P < 0.05$).

6. Clinical results

The deep tendon reflex polyneuropathy patients have a significantly decreased reflex when compared with all differential diagnosis ($P < 0.05$, Duncan). Regarding the presence of atrophy when all cases are compared with the WHS, there is no significant difference. In terms of hand complaints, polyneuropathy has a higher complaint score (1.3 ± 1.33; $P < 0.05$) when compared with the healthy normal group. However, the WHS (3.00 ± 0.00) and CTS (3.00 ± 0.00) groups exhibit an increase in hand complaints when compared with both the healthy and polyneuropathy.

7. Other comorbid diseases in the WHS

In terms of diabetes mellitus, hypertension, cardiovascular diseases, hyperlipidemia, cigarette smoking, and the presence of atrophy, when all cases are compared with the WHS, there is no significant difference according to Fisher exact test.

8. Differential diagnosis in the WHS

The use of a vibrating tool by the patients and the presence of a nervous system disease, such as polyneuropathy, CTS, or hand-arm vibration syndrome (HAVS). The diagnosis of distal axonal sensory polyneuropathy is extracted from nerve conduction work-up reports based on the presence of bilateral, symmetric, and distal lower and upper extremity neuropathic pain. The motor nerves are unaffected, and there is no muscle weakness in this condition. Only the hands experience neuropathic pain in the WHS, while there is neuropathic pain in both the feet and hands in the polyneuropathy. Sensory nerve conduction work-ups of the median, ulnar, and sural nerves are widely used in the electrodiagnosis of sensory polyneuropathy. The long nerves are most commonly affected by polyneuropathy. Thus, the sural sensory nerve action potential (SNAP) amplitude is likely the most useful parameter for differentiating normal subjects from those with distal sensory polyneuropathy. Even the sural SNAP is most sensitive in the diagnosis of early distal sensory polyneuropathy. The sural nerve results are significantly affected in the polyneuropathy, while the WHS have normal sural nerve conduction work-ups.

Several diseases affect the nerves of the hand, the most common being CTS, which is caused by median nerves in the carpal tunnels becoming stuck. It is characterized by neuropathic complaints in the first four fingers and the palm of the hand. Its symptoms manifest usually during rest hours or nighttime, and the cases identified in the WHS are similar in that regard. This means the entirety of their hand and the fingers have neuropathic pain. Women are more commonly affected by CTS, and rheumatism, pregnancy, and diabetes are among the known risk factors for CTS. All of the WHS cases are men, and they have no known CTS risk factors. Characteristic electrophysiological findings of CTS include a progressively delayed sensory peak latency, and amplitude becomes smaller in the median nerve. In medium cases, similar findings appear in the motor nerves. In advanced cases, SNAP and compound muscle action potential (CMAP) values decrease, which means that in CTS, a delayed distal latency and decrease in velocity are pronounced in the median nerve. The ulnar nerve conduction work-ups in CTS are normal. In the WHS, according to the normal, distal latency and velocity are close to normal, but both the median sensory and ulnar sensory nerve amplitudes are decreased. Motor values are completely normal.

Guyon canal and cubital tunnel entrapment neuropathies can cause neuropathic pain, as well [8], but neuropathic pain is seen only in the ulnar nerve tract. In nerve conduction studies, distal latency and velocity are affected in the ulnar nerve. In all of the cases herein, neuropathic pain is identified in every region of the hand. Not only the ulnar nerve but also the median nerve is affected.

The mechanical energy created by vibrating tools, which enters the body through the fingers or palms, is called hand-arm vibration. These tools are generally used in the production, stone working, mining, construction, agriculture, and forestry sectors. HAVS is a clinical condition that occurs after exposure to hand-arm vibration. Symptoms of HAVS include numbness, pain, and reduced dexterity, strength, and sensation in the hands. In HAVS, the peripheral and central nervous systems are affected, which can lead to vascular, bone and joint, and tendon and muscle diseases. There is a direct correlation between the disease and the magnitude and duration of hand-arm vibration and cold temperatures. In the cases here in, no vibrating tools are used by the patients, but they engage in taxing labor using their hands (using such tools as a sledgehammer, hammer, saw, and carry stones). It is argued that the usage of beta-blockers and cigarettes and a decrease in blood circulation due to exposure to the cold lead to an increase in HAVS symptoms. According to the anamnesis of the patients in the WHS, their symptoms do not change in cold temperatures or after smoking. CTS is often observed in people with HAVS who engage in breaking stones, plating, and forestry. This means that HAVS itself can cause CTS. Electrophysiological studies aimed at defining the nature of a vibration injury have provided conflicting results. Usually, electrophysiological findings related to HAVS are similar to those related to CTS, and the effect on velocity is pronounced. These conditions can be seen together often.

The ulnar nerve is rarely affected in HAVS, but both the ulnar and median nerves are affected in the WHS. Especially, the ulnar nerve is affected. In HAVS, slowed sensory nerve conduction velocities are often observed in the hands. In the WHS, especially, the amplitude is low without being greatly affected by speed and latency. In vibration-associated neuropathies, conceivable target structures could be peripheral sensory receptors, large or thin myelinated nerve fibers, and small-caliber, non-myelinated C fibers. Pathological studies by cutaneous biopsy have demonstrated demyelinating neuropathy in the digital nerves of individuals with HAVS [5–8].

9. Treatment options

In treatment of polyneuropathy, the primary goal in the evaluation of neuropathy is to identify the etiology and if possible treat the underlying cause. Medical causes such as diabetes mellitus, renal insufficiency, hypothyroidism, vitamin B-12 deficiency, and Guillain-Barré syndrome need specific treatments. But, there is no specific treatment for many chronic neuropathies such as chronic idiopathic axonal polyneuropathy or the hereditary neuropathies. One of the most limiting symptoms is neuropathic pain. The neuropathic pain can be effectively treated with an algorithmic approach. In the WHS, there is no specific treatment yet. However, I gave 75 mg pregabalin.

10. Conclusion and future directions

The WHS is a new disorder. It is also an occupational disease. I think that a significant number of patients as this should not to be underestimated in the general population. We only considered it previously as a sensory polyneuropathy in upper limbs. For this reason, we need to examine it more in detail from the etiopathogenesis to its treatment. This disorder is suggested to serve as a resource for patients, healthcare professionals, and members of the neurology community at large.

Author details

Gökhan Özdemir
Department of Neurology, Selcuk University Medical Faculty, Konya, Turkey

*Address all correspondence to: noro.ozdemir@gmail.com

References

[1] Özdemir G. Working hand syndrome. A new definition of non-classified polyneuropathy condition. Medicine. 2017;**96**(25):e7235

[2] Hanewinckel R, Drenthen J, van Oijen M, Hofman A, van Doorn PA, Ikram MA. Prevalence of polyneuropathy in the general middle-aged and elderly population. Neurology. 2016;**87**:1892-1898

[3] England JD, Gronseth GS, Franklin G, et al. Practice parameter: Evaluation of distal symmetric polyneuropathy: Role of laboratory and genetic testing (an evidence-based review): Report of the American Academy of Neurology, American Association of Neuromuscular and Electrodiagnostic Medicine, and American Academy of Physical Medicine and Rehabilitation. Neurology. 2009;**72**:185-192

[4] Rosenberg NR, Portegies P, deVisser M, Vermeulen M. Diagnostic investigation of patients with chronic polyneuropathy: Evaluation of a clinical guideline. Journal of Neurology, Neurosurgery, and Psychiatry. 2001;**71**:205-209

[5] Deutsche Gesellschaft für Neurologie: S1 Leitlinie Diagnostik bei Polyneuropathien. www.dgn.org/leitlinien/2331-ll-44-2012-diagnostik-beipolyneuropathien [Accessed: December 8, 2017]

[6] Sommer C, Üçeyler N. Small-fiber-neuropathien. Klinische Neurophysiologie. 2017;**48**:63-72

[7] Prior R, van Helleputte L, Benoy V, van den Bosch L. Defective axonal transport: A common pathological mechanism in inherited and acquired peripheral neuropathies. Neurobiology of Disease. 2017;**105**:300-320

[8] Beghi E, Monticelli ML. Chronic symmetric symptomatic polyneuropathy in the elderly: A field screening investigation of risk factors for polyneuropathy in two Italian communities. Italian General Practitioner Study Group (IGPST). Journal of Clinical Epidemiology. 1998 Aug;**51**(8):697-702

Section 3

Management and New Clinical Applications

Chapter 5

Platelet-Rich Plasma for Injured Peripheral Nerves: Biological Repair Process and Clinical Application Guidelines

Mikel Sánchez, Ane Garate, Ane Miren Bilbao, Jaime Oraa, Fernando Yangüela, Pello Sánchez, Jorge Guadilla, Beatriz Aizpurua, Juan Azofra, Nicolás Fiz and Diego Delgado

Abstract

Platelet-rich plasma (PRP) is a biological therapy that uses the patient's own blood to obtain products with a higher platelet concentration than in blood. It provides a transient fibrin scaffold as a controlled drug delivery system of growth factors suitable for regenerative medicine. PRP has been used as medical strategy to treat diverse types of injuries in the field of orthopedics, including peripheral nerve lesions. In vitro and in vivo studies showed the neuroprotective, neurogenic and neuroinflammatory modulator effect of PRP. In addition, it has been demonstrated clinically that PRP infiltrations improve clinical symptoms and enhance the sensory and motor functional nerve muscle unit recovery. Potential effects of PRP could be applied in treatments for neuropathies, as conservative treatment by means of nerve ultrasound-guided infiltrations or as biological adjuvant during surgery.

Keywords: platelet-rich plasma, growth factors, neuropathies, intraneural injection, perineural injection, US-guided injection

1. Introduction

Diverse health conditions or traumatic injuries such as accidents, stretching or compressions may cause damage on nerves. Some options to treat these damages are oral drugs, steroid injections, physical therapy or surgical interventions. Probably, nerve autografts or direct tension-free microsurgical repairs are the most common treatments aimed to enhance the intrinsic regenerative potential of injured axons. However, they do not recreate the suitable cellular and molecular microenvironment of peripheral nerve repair.

To overcome this drawback, new therapeutic strategies have been developed for these conditions, using various models of nerve injuries. In vitro models of neuronal survival include cell cultures or tissue engineering advances, whereas in vivo models involve lesions in peripheral nerves of many species. These studies lead to develop new strategies based on tissue engineering approaches through molecular intervention and scaffolding, and platelet-rich plasma (PRP) represents one of these promising biological strategies. Large number of studies provides evidence for PRP application in musculoskeletal disorders and orthopedics. Applications include treatments of chondropathy, osteoarthritis, tendinopathy, muscle or ligament tear, acute and chronic soft tissue injuries, as well as enhancement of healing after bone or tissue reconstruction [1]. In addition to its positive effects on the healing of many types of tissues, recent studies reported the promising effects of PRP on nerve regeneration [2]. Indeed, several preclinical and clinical studies have proved the neuroprotective, neurogenic and neuroinflammatory properties of this therapy. Moreover, pain reduction, function improvement and nerve-muscle unit recovery have been demonstrated after applying diverse PRP formulations including liquid and scaffold form. This chapter is intended to overview the advances made on this specific field, focusing on the concept of PRP, its biological effects on nerve repair and its clinical application.

2. Platelet-rich plasma

PRP is an autologous product with a higher platelet concentration than in blood. It consists of a pool of bioactive mediators including growth factors (GF), cytokines, microparticles and others from patient's own blood. Currently, there are several methods and commercial devices to achieve PRP, obtaining a diversity of products including autologous conditioned plasma, platelet-enriched plasma, platelet-rich concentrate, autogenous platelet gel, platelet releasate, platelet rich in GFs and others [3]. Some parameters and characteristics such as platelet concentration, the presence of leucocytes or the fibrin architecture may vary depending on the method or device employed to obtain these refined products. The processing technique to achieve PRP mostly consists of a blood collection in the presence of an anticoagulant followed by centrifugation. This centrifugation separates the blood components with the aim of discarding substances considered as not usable such as red blood cells and concentrating the elements with therapeutic potential, for instance fibrinogen/fibrin, platelets or GF, with or without leukocytes (**Figure 1**). Before its administration, an activating factor such as thrombin or calcium is added to the platelet concentrate to promote platelet degranulation and exocytosis of the factors stored in the cytoplasmic granules [4].

Indeed, the potential effect of PRP is closely related with the release of bioactive molecules stored in alpha granules of platelets after its activation with the activating factor [5]. Platelet-derived growth factor (PDGF), transforming growth factor (TGF-β), epidermal growth factor (EGF), insulin-like growth factor (IGF-1), hepatocyte growth factor (HGF), basic fibroblasts growth factor (FGF) and vascular endothelial growth factor (VEGF) are some of the key proteins associated with the acceleration of healing process, since they modulate angiogenesis, remodel the extracellular matrix (ECM) and affect the recruitment, proliferation and differentiation of stem cells [6]. The wide variety of elements found in platelet granules act synergistically under normal physiological conditions on local cells to promote wound healing. On the other hand, plasma activation also promotes the polymerization of fibrinogen into a three-dimensional fibrin scaffold (**Figure 1**), maintaining the bioactive mediators trapped through fibrin heparin sulfate-binding domains [1]. This biocompatible and biodegradable scaffold provides plastic-elastic stiffness and generates GF gradients that are essential cues for cell proliferation, differentiation, migration and correct orientation in the nascent tissue [7]. When fibrinolysis begins, a gradual, sustained release of GF and other biomolecules occurs, in contrast to a bolus delivery modality. Thus, this technology provides a fibrin scaffold as a controlled drug delivery system of GF suitable for regenerative medicine [8].

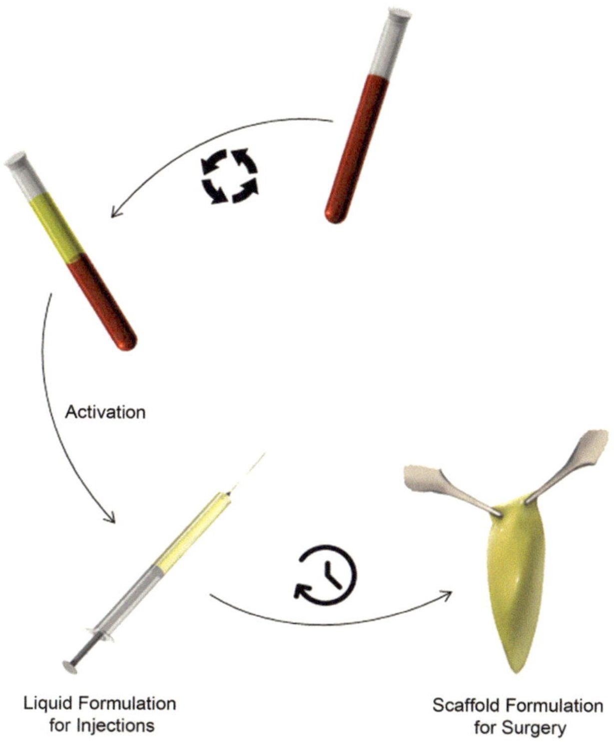

Figure 1.
Platelet-rich plasma formulation. After withdrawing a small volume of venous blood in tubes containing anticoagulant, these are centrifuged in order to separate the blood components. The plasma fraction located just above the red blood cells is collected including or not leukocytes. PRP is activated adding thrombin or calcium to promote platelet degranulation and exocytosis of GF. This liquid formulation is used to conduct PRP injections. If after activation, the waiting time is prolonged, fibrin formation is achieved, obtaining a scaffold for applying in surgery.

Due to its primarily autologous origin and relatively noninvasive collection technique, the risks of injection or immune rejection associated with PRP are minimized, making this biological therapy a powerful tool for its application on diverse medical fields. Thus, this strategy has been employed as a biological adjuvant in peripheral nerve injuries and neuropathies, enhancing the sensory and motor functional nerve-muscle unit recovery [9]. In cases of nontraumatic peripheral injuries such as compression, adhesion and/or fibrotic postsurgical side effects, PRP may help diminish undesirable consequences such as denervated organ atrophy and fibrotic scars.

3. Biological effects of PRP on nerve regeneration

Among therapeutic alternatives to restore damaged nerves, PRP is gaining attention, since it provides the infiltrated environment with a pool of GF inducing healing and regeneration of the tissue. Nerve growth factor (NGF), brain-derived neurotrophic factor (BDNF) and PDGF are some of PRP components that can improve nerve regeneration. However, a sustained delivery of several GFs is not the unique constituent of PRP effect on nerve regeneration. Indeed, in vitro and in vivo evidence suggests that the biomolecules transmitted by PRP are instrumental agents that act as key drivers of full nerve functional recovery, offering a new possibility for nerve regeneration (**Figure 2**).

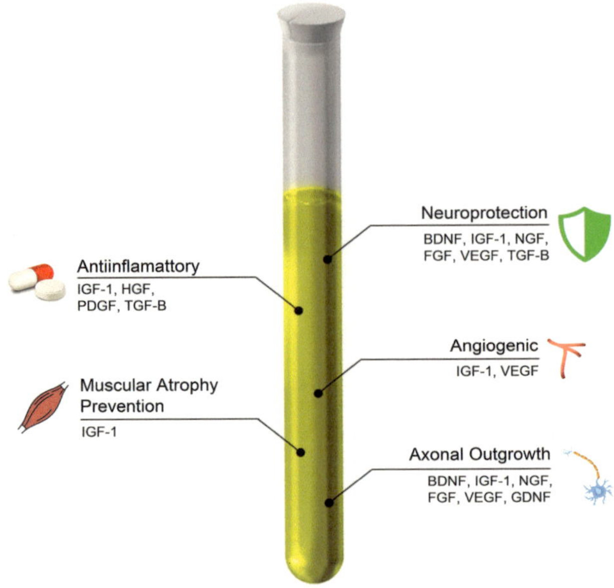

Figure 2.
Effects of PRP on nerve repair. Biomolecules and GF participate jointly and synergistically in several biological processes involved in nerve regeneration.

3.1 Neuroprotection and prevention of cell apoptosis

An important factor that plays a critical role in many functions within the nervous system including neurogenesis and neuroprotective function is BDNF. One of the most important benefits that this biomolecule offers is its ability to inhibit neuronal and glial apoptosis after traumatic injury. A work carried out by Koda et al. proved that BDNF suppressed in a dose-dependent manner anoikis of Schwann cells (SC), which are able to promote axonal regeneration and functional recovery [10]. This effect is based on the activation or transdifferentiation of SCs, a drastic modification of the phenotype of this cell type that takes place after the disruption of the regeneration unit by the noxious agent. Macrophages will collaborate with the activated SCs clearing the myelin and other tissue debris. Moreover, these SCs come into direct contact with resident fibroblasts accumulated in large numbers at the site of injury, influencing SC migration and transdifferentiation. In another work, Wang et al. found that mesenchymal stem cells (MSCs) transfected with Ad-BDNF enhance the expression of BDNF, recovering brain damage. They suggest that BDNF-MSCs have a potential protective effect against neuron death by apoptosis [11]. In another study, Zurita et al. enriched PRP fibrin scaffolds with bone marrow stromal cells with BDNF, NGF and retinoic acid, enhancing cell survival and differentiation into the neural phenotype [12]. Another GF related with neuronal and Schwann cell survival is IGF-1. This factor acts as neurotrophic factor for sensory, motor and sympathetic neurons to promote growth cone motility and prevent apoptosis [13]. It has also been proved that neurons express PDGF receptors, and the function related with this GF on nerve injury also involves the survival for Schwann cells with trophic activity on neurons [14]. Other substances such as NGF, FGF, VEGF and TGF-β presented in PRP have shown to exert an antiapoptotic and neuroprotective effect on diverse cell types such as MSCs, neurons, Schwann cells and human neural stem cells [15].

3.2 Anti-inflammatory effects

Anti-inflammatory action of PRP is associated with an inhibition of nuclear transcription factor-kB (NF-kB) pathway, which was observed after culturing astrocytes with PRP supernatants [16]. Some of the GFs such as HGF, IGF-1, PDGF and TGF-β delivered in a sustained way after PRP infiltrations are closely related with these effects [15]. TGF-β also affects cellular behavior, the neurite outgrowth and glial scar formation [17]. Outcomes from an in vivo study further suggested that TGF-β coordinated with adipose-derived MSCs enhanced nerve regeneration affecting the host's immune response and reducing inflammation [15].

PRP injections have been associated with a decrease of proinflammatory substances such as nitric oxide, cyclooxygenase and tumor necrosis factor expressed in the brain [16]. In addition, PRP is able to block Ab-induced upregulation of proinflammatory cytokine production, and this capacity was correlated with a prevention of the decrease in several synaptic proteins.

3.3 Angiogenic properties

Among the substances that PRP contains, VEGF is one of the most angiogenic factors. It stimulates proliferation and migration of endothelial cells, formation of new blood vessels and enhances vascular permeability. This action is conducted by transmembrane receptors found in neural tissue, especially on growth cones of sprouting axons and Schwann cells [18]. VEGF can act as a neurotrophic factor by promoting Schwann cell proliferation and neurite outgrowth and enhance nerve survival [19]. However, despite the evidence that PRP promotes angiogenesis in tendon, muscle and bone and the crucial role that blood vessels play as trackers of the axonal growth cones across the injury site, there is lack of studies assessing angiogenesis in nerve repair. Borselli et al. showed that an injectable scaffold loaded with VEGF and IGF-1 accelerated regeneration of damaged neuromuscular junction innervation together with an enhancement of angiogenesis in an ischemic limb rodent model [20]. Another study demonstrated that vein graft filled with PRP provides an earlier and more prominent neoangiogenesis than sciatic nerve gaps treated with nerve autograft alone [21]. The fibrin obtained after PRP activation provides a permissive and robust 3D matrix for angiogenesis. In fact, autologous fibrin matrix is the best tailored transient scaffold for tissue regeneration where complex morphogenetic processes for tissue regeneration take place, including angiogenesis, cell migration and proliferation [22].

3.4 Enhancing axonal outgrowth capacity

Schwann cells provide bioactive substrates for axonal migration and they release neurotrophic factors able to regulate axonal outgrowth. An optimal proliferation and viability may affect the rapid regeneration of injured peripheral nerves. PRP might allow the sprouting of growth cones since they promote survival, proliferation and differentiation of Schwann cells. In that sense, Zheng et al. showed a dose-dependent effect of PRP on the proliferation, migration and neurotrophic function in rat Schwann cells cultured with PRP [23]. The significant role played by GF within the PRP has also been highlighted in a rat brain-spinal cord cocultured system, where the addition of PRP supernatant promoted an increase in the size and number of axons. This positive effect was significantly suppressed by the addition of antibodies against IGF-1 and VEGF [24].

Solid form of PRP also demonstrated its positive effect on both axonal myelination and its density enhancement. Ye et al. fabricated tissue-engineered nerves based on poly (lactic-co-glycolic acid) conduit using PRP gel for suspension of Schwann cell–like cells. PRP group presented superior functionality in both nerve conduction velocity and compound muscle action potential. They suggest that PRP gel plays a dual role: first, the fibrin network as matrix for regenerative cell incorporation, and second, biomolecules that improve the biological environment stimulating the regenerative processes of nerve fibers [25]. Indeed, the PRP bioactive proteins initiate and control the healing cascade of nerve fibers. Increasing the concentration of these bioactive proteins such as TGF-β, PDGF and IGF-1 could accelerate healing of the regenerating nerve fibers [26]. Other studies realized in rabbits after implantation of PRP together with Schwann cells [27] reported beneficial effects on axonal counts, myelination and electrophysiological parameters. Cho et al. observed considerably increased expression of neurotrophic factors such as BDNF, NGF, FGF and Glial cell–derived neurotrophic factor (GDNF) after PRP injection in guinea pigs with facial nerve transection, suggesting that PRP and MSCs act as a source of neurotrophic factors. They also could prove an enhancement of axon counts and myelination in the groups treated with PRP [27]. An inside-out vein autograft filled with PRP was used to bridge a 10-mm-long sciatic nerve defect in rats [21]. The axon diameter, the number of myelinated axons and myelin sheath were significantly superior when vein autograph was filled with PRP. In another rat model, they used platelet-rich fibrin (PRF) as a filler of silicon nerve guidance. Animals treated with PRP improved functional recovery and showed a superior sciatic functional index compared to nontreated animals [28].

3.5 Dampening the denervated target muscle atrophy

The acceleration of axonal growth can prevent muscle atrophy, since it reduces the time to establish a connection between the sprouting axon and target muscle [29]. PRP applications induce an earlier axonal regeneration and functional recovery, which also can have a consequence reducing the target muscle atrophy. In the work carried out by Sánchez et al., they could observe this positive effect since nerves repaired with intraneural infiltrations of PRP were associated with lower muscle atrophy and an earlier electrophysiological recovery [30]. In some peripheral nerve injuries such as carpal tunnel syndrome or fibrotic postsurgical side effects, the main pathological agent is compression, adhesion and/or fibrosis. The use of PRP may additionally avoid or at least diminish denervated organ atrophy and undesirable fibrotic scars, thereby accelerating the functional recovery of the nerve-muscle unit, due to its antifibrotic effects [24, 31]. Intramuscular injection of PRP 24 hours after the induction of limb ischemia in mice mitigated fibrosis and muscle atrophy [32]. These results are in agreement with the reduction of atrophy in denervated muscle reported when muscle was infiltrated with cells [33], effects suggested to be mediated by IGF-1 [34].

4. Clinical guidelines for the application of platelet-rich plasma in injured peripheral nerves: from bench to bedside

Although the biological effects described previously mean a promising therapeutic tool, the success to achieve optimal clinical results lies in several factors such as PRP preparation, dosage and application protocols.

4.1 PRP preparation

Physicians face a large number of systems to obtain PRP and therefore different types of final products. These depend on variables such as platelet concentration, the presence or absence of leukocytes and the exogenous activation of PRP. Although there is still no consensus on which is the best product to use in orthopedic pathologies, according to preclinical research and our experience, we suggest choosing a product with specific characteristics.

An excessive number of platelets could not only suppress the therapeutic action of PRP but also inhibit the tissue repair process. PRP with excess platelet concentration had negative influence over cellular responses such as proliferation, viability or differentiation [35]. Thus, it seems that a concentration of platelet slightly higher than blood is suitable to achieve an optimal response. The presence of leukocytes in PRP products is more controversial. While in tissues like cartilage the scale tips in favor of the PRP without leukocytes, in other applications, it is not clear. The presence of leukocytes fosters the nuclear NF-κB p65 protein expression, which is key in the activation of cellular inflammation, and oddly enough, it is inhibited by PRP [36]. Finally, and although platelets within PRP can be activated endogenously by tissue collagen, we recommend the previous activation in an exogenous way, which is carried out by adding calcium to PRP. As calcium was chelated during blood extraction to avoid coagulation, we restore the levels of it in PRP preventing hypocalcemia in nerve environment during infiltration. The activation triggers the formation of a fibrin 3D liquid scaffold that spreads over the tissue, delivering GF in a control manner. After activation, PRP must be injected immediately during the following 10 minutes. Without activating, it can be stored for 3–4 hours without losing its efficacy. PRP can be applied also as a fibrin scaffold for using in surgery. This scaffold is obtained in the same way as the liquid formulation, except that after its activation, the waiting time before its use is prolonged until the formation of the fibrin scaffold (**Figure 1**). Despite these recommendations, it is in the hands of the professional who applies PRP to choose the best suitable type, and following the manufacturer's protocol is advisable to obtain an optimal product.

4.2 Conducting nerve infiltrations

In order to achieve the biological effects described in Section 3, PRP must be administered in an adequate manner to reach the target tissue and cells that are key elements in nerve repair process such as Schwann cells. However, they are in the innermost compartment of the nerve, inside the fascicles that enclose the axons covered by the myelin sheaths, and getting to them is a major issue. For many years, nerve infiltration has been and still is a controversial point for physicians and medical specialists. Although a possible cause of nerve lesions during an injection is the ischemic damage due to increased pressure inside the nerve, the most likely reason is the neurotoxicity of the injected drug such as corticosteroids or local anesthetics. Several studies demonstrated that the injuries caused to the nerve after infiltrations were because of the injected drug or its dose, and not because of the physical act of infiltrating [37].

The compartment of the nerve where the injection is performed is also a sensitive point to consider. Although some studies recommend avoiding intraneural injection due to high risk of nerve lesion [38], it is necessary to be more precise in this description. We must distinguish between extrafascicular and intrafascicular injection, the former being safe and without any evidence of nerve injury [39]. In contrast, some studies conclude that the main cause of neurologic injury is the intrafascicular injections [40]. Brierley et al. studied the progression of nerve lesions in some diseases like tetanus or poliomyelitis using radioactive phosphorus. He found that the phosphorus reached the blood stream, the cerebrospinal fluid and the nervous system when the needle penetrated into the fasciculus, thus being an intrafascicular injection [41]. Diffusion studies of PRP into the nerve carried out by our group showed that PRP previously stained with methylene blue was accumulated around the perineurium after intraneural but not intrafascicular injections, without reaching inside the fascicle through the perineurium [2] (**Figure 3**).

4.3 Conservative treatment with US-guided infiltrations of PRP

Throughout this section, we will describe the procedures to perform US-guided infiltrations of PRP in some nerves susceptible to peripheral lesions, namely median nerve (**Figure 4**), ulnar nerve (**Figure 5**) and common peroneal nerve (**Figure 6**). The infiltrations of the nerves mentioned in this section share a large number of key points, which are described below. The details of each nerve are shown in **Table 1**.

4.3.1 Key points for common US-guided neural infiltrations

a. Preparation of the sterile field is required to maintain aseptic conditions throughout the treatment. The skin covering the affected nerve and the transducer of the US machine must be prepared following standard asepsis protocols.

b. Prior to the infiltrations, the nerve must be located by means of US in the pertinent areas. During this step, the US probe can be used in a long- as well as short-axis in respect to the nerve so that its examination can be as accurate as possible.

c. In the course of PRP injections, the needle is placed parallel to the US probe, and consequently its orientation in respect to the nerve has influence on the PRP diffusion. With the transductor in the long-axis in respect to the nerve, the needle is introduced almost parallel to it, spreading PRP along the nerve. If the US probe is placed in the short-axis, the needle is inserted at right angles to the nerve increasing the risk of injury axon. The spread is less than in the previous case, especially when the diameter of the nerve is large. However, this approach allows better visualization of the tissue. Therefore, we recommend using the US transductor that achieves a balance between diffusion and nerve visualization.

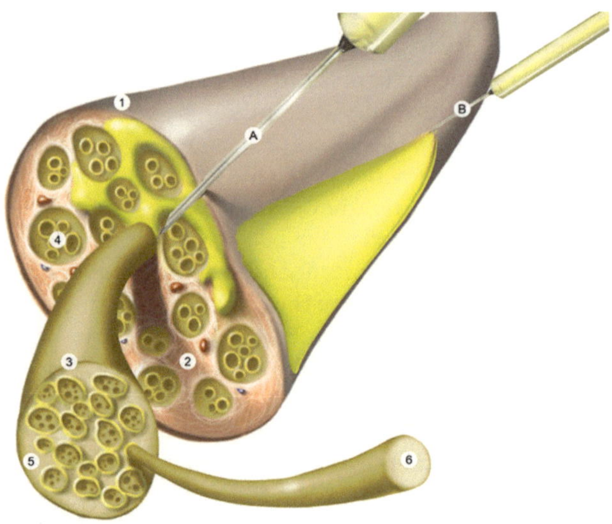

Figure 3.
Nerve infiltration. During the procedure, two injections are conducted. First, intraneural infiltration (A) reaches the intrafascicular epineurium (2) and next, the perineural infiltration (B) is performed around the nerve. 1 = epineurium; 2 = intrafascicular epineurium; 3 = perineurium; 4 = fascicle; 5 = endoneurium; 6 = axon covered by myelin.

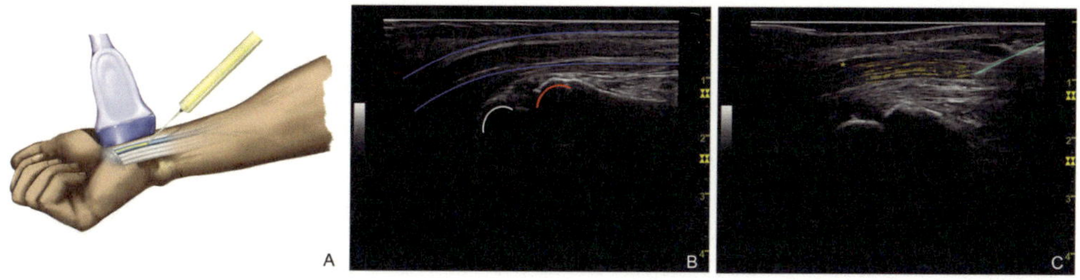

Figure 4.
Median nerve infiltration. The median nerve is located by means of US in the area of the wrist (A). Under US control with the probe placed in long-axis, the nerve (blue) is observed above the epiphyses of the distal radius (red) and lunate bone (white) (B). The needle (green) is inserted in distal-proximal direction, and PRP is injected in an intraneural (yellow) and perineural way (asterisk) (C).

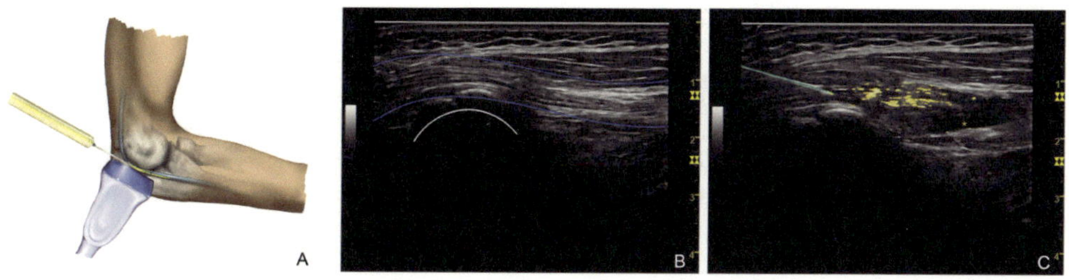

Figure 5.
Ulnar nerve infiltration. The ulnar nerve is located by means of US in the area of the elbow (A). Under US control with the probe placed in long-axis, the nerve (blue) is observed above the epicondyle (white) (B). The needle (green) is inserted in distal-proximal direction, and PRP is injected in an intraneural (yellow) and perineural way (asterisk) (C). In this case, the injection could be conducted in proximal-distal direction if the access is difficult.

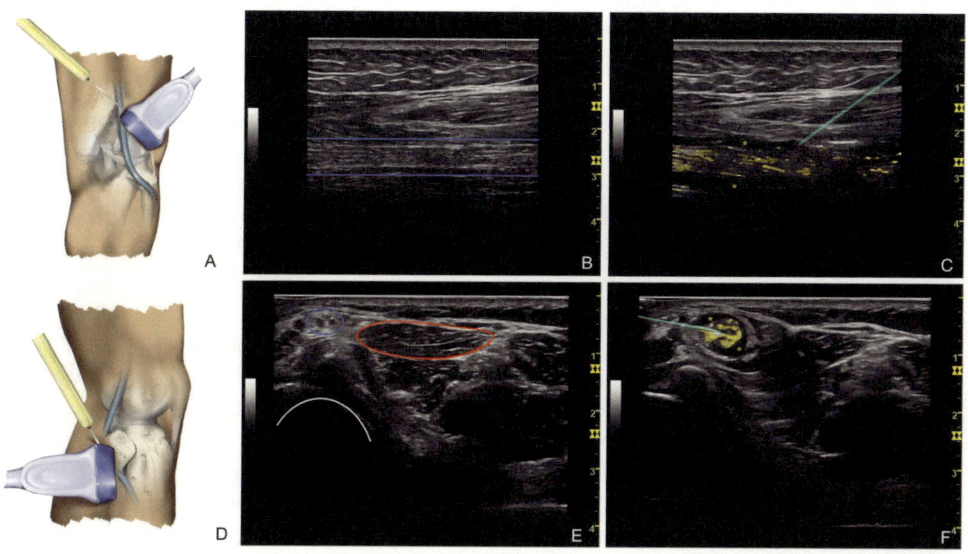

Figure 6.
Common peroneal nerve infiltration. Two approaches are possible to infiltrate common peroneal nerve. In the first approach, the nerve (blue) is located by US above the popliteal fossa with the US transductor in the long axis (A and B). In the second approach, the nerve is located in the lateral side of the knee (D). With the probe placed in the short axis, the nerve (blue) is observed above the peroneal head (white) and close to tibialis anterior muscle (red) (E). In both cases, the needle (green) is inserted in proximal-distal direction, injecting PRP in an intraneural (yellow) and perineural way (asterisk) (C and F).

	Median nerve	Ulnar nerve	Common peroneal nerve	
			Approach 1	Approach 2
Indication	Compressive neuropathies such as CTS	Compressive neuropathies such as UTS	Nerve lesions associated to knee injuries	
Patient position	Sitting with the arm flexed and supported on flat surface	Supine position	Prone position	Lateral position over the healthy side
Limb position	Supination, the palm of the hand facing upward	Pronation, with the elbow lightly flexed and on a padded support	Extended leg	Lightly knee flexion and on a padded support
Infiltration area	Wrist, around the distal area of the radius	Behind medial epicondyle, into cubital tunnel	Back of the thigh, around the popliteal fossa above the knee	Lateral knee area around the peroneal head
Syringe	Luer-Lok, 3 mL	Luer-Lok, 3 mL	Luer-Lok, 5 mL	Luer-Lok, 5 mL
Needle	23 G/25 mm	23 G/25 mm	21 G/50 mm	21 G/50 mm
Direction	Proximal-distal	Both	Proximal-distal	Proximal-distal
Intraneural vol.	2 mL	3 mL	3 mL	3 mL
Perineural vol.	4 mL	6 mL	6 mL	6 mL

CTS, carpal tunnel syndrome; UTS, ulnar tunnel syndrome; Vol, volume.

Table 1.
Characteristics of platelet-rich plasma US-guided infiltrations for different nerves.

d. The proximal-distal direction is preferable so that PRP spreads through the nerve. In some cases as injections into ulnar nerve, the direction can also be from distal to proximal zone if the injured area is unapproachable.

e. Both intraneural and perineural injections are performed during the treatment. Activated PRP is injected softly and without rough movements of the needle to prevent nerve damage. As the PRP volume required for both infiltrations can exceed the capacity of the syringe, changes of syringes for loading them with PRP can be done without removing the needle from the injection site, thus avoiding repeated punctures.

f. Firstly, it is advisable to perform the intraneural infiltration with the needle reaching the intrafascicular epineurium of the nerve. During intraneural injection, PRP shows some hyperechoic signals under US control within the nerve.

g. Once intraneural injection is accomplished, the needle is gently retreated placing it just above the nerve to conduct the perineural injection around the nerve. The adjacent tissue to the nerve is detached when perineural infiltration is performed, appearing as a hypoechoic signal. This infiltration entails a hydrodissection that reduces nerve entrapment through a mechanical effect [42].

h. The dosage of these treatments is determined by the nerve size to be infiltrated, which is detailed in each case (**Table 1**). In all cases, it is recommended to carry out two treatments, with an interval of two between both visits.

i. The follow-up is conducted 4 weeks after finishing the treatment. Clinical examination is required in order to observe improvement in clinical parameters such as pain and paresthesia. Depending on the patient's condition, we will follow different recommendation:

   - If the patient shows a significant improvement, no intervention will be performed. Six weeks after clinical follow-up, an electromyography (EMG) will be conducted to evaluate the state of the nerve and assess possible actions.

   - When the patient evolution has flat-lined or is not enough, neural infiltrations with PRP will be repeated again.

   - In case the patient has not experienced any improvement, infiltrations of PRP will be discarded and other treatment alternatives will be considered. An EMG study should be performed in the third month.

4.3.2 Subgluteal sciatic compression

a. PRP infiltrations into this nerve are indicated for compressive neuropathies such as pyramidal syndrome or deep gluteal syndrome.

b. The patient is placed as in the case of the sciatic nerve approach, namely in prone decubitus on a flat surface.

c. By means of US control, the nerve is located at the level popliteal fossa, and then the nerve path is followed until gluteal fold, where PRP injection in distal-proximal direction is conducted. If the nerve can be located in a more proximal area, the infiltration can also be performed following the proximal-distal direction.

d. The injection is conducted with 10 mL in a syringe fitted with an 18 G and 75 mm needle and US probe placed in the long axis.

e. Four ml of activated PRP is administered during intraneural infiltration and 8 mL of activated PRP is infiltrated around the nerve.

4.3.3 Neuromas

Traumatic neuroma follows different forms of nerve injury often as a result of surgery. They occur at the end of injured nerve fibers as a form of ineffective, unregulated nerve regeneration. Due to the peculiarities of these neuropathies, the volume of the product, the type of syringes and needles to infiltrate the PRP will largely depend on the nerve where the neuroma is located, which was described above. In addition, not only an intraneural and a perineural injection into neuroma are conducted but also in the proximal nerve close to the neuroma.

4.4 PRP as adjuvant in surgery

In many cases, surgical interventions are required for the treatment of neuropathies. Among these, the neurolysis is a standard procedure to separate the nerve from the surrounding tissues and try to solve problems related to compression and entrapment. In these cases, the use of PRP as a therapeutic adjuvant during surgery can stimulate and accelerate nerve recovery. Next, both endoscopic (**Figure 7**) and open neurolysis (**Figure 8**) of a median nerve are explained. Neurolysis in other nerves will be done in the same way but adapting to the particularities of each nerve.

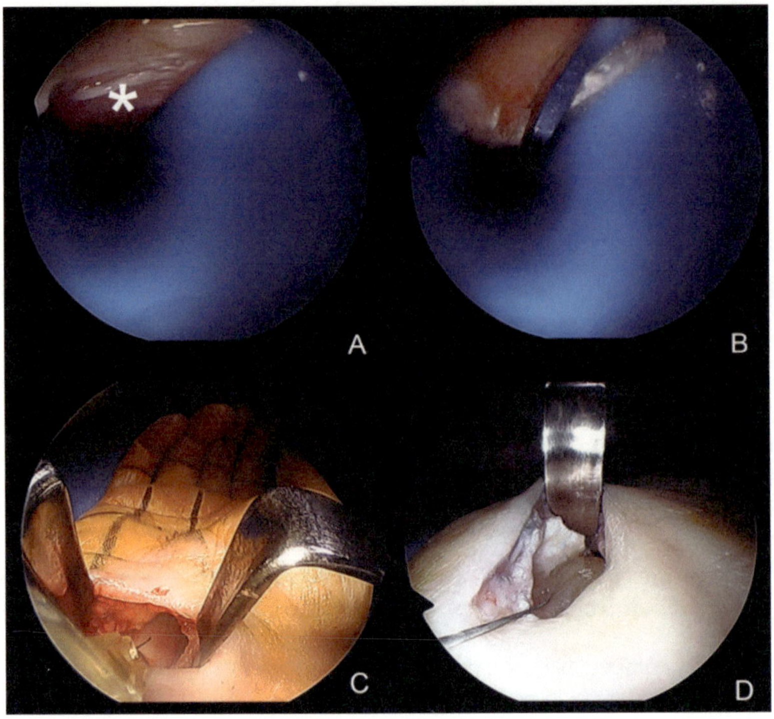

Figure 7.
Endoscopic neurolysis of median nerve. Endoscopic camera and cannula are introduced into the wrist (A). Carpal ligament (asterisk) is dissected and cut (B). PRP is infiltrated into the nerve (C) and a fibrin clot is placed between the nerve and the ligament (D).

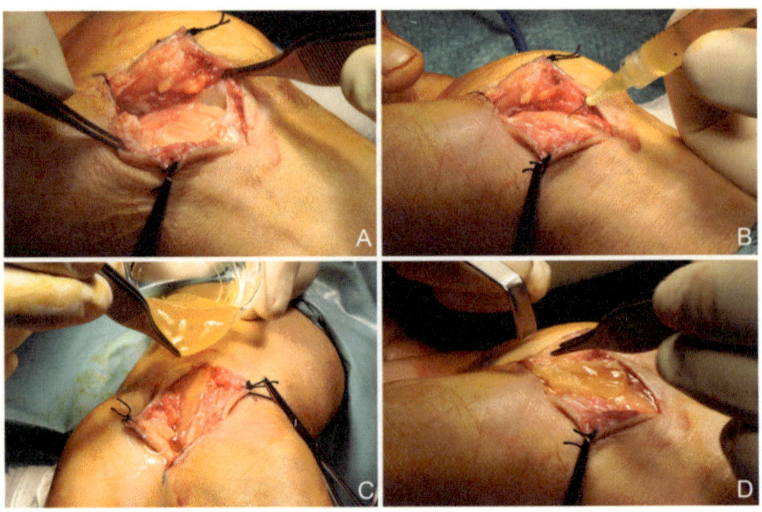

Figure 8.
Open neurolysis of median nerve. Median nerve and the transverse carpal ligament are observed after incision (A). Once median nerve is released, PRP is injected (B). Finally, fibrin membrane (C) is placed between the nerve and the ligament (D).

4.4.1 Endoscopic neurolysis

a. After performing a small incision at the level of wrist crease, a cannula is introduced in order to observe structures in the wrist as the transverse carpal ligament with an endoscopic camera.

b. When the transverse carpal ligament is located and dissected, it is cut with endoscopic knife so that the median nerve is released.

c. Once the ligament is sectioned and nerve released, 2 mL of PRP is infiltrated into the nerve from the incision made for arthroscopy with a 30 G needle. A fibrin clot is placed in the open carpal tunnel before suturing.

4.4.2 Open surgical neurolysis

a. An incision at the level of wrist crease is conducted. The incision must be large enough to observe and access to the median nerve and the transverse carpal ligament.

b. Next, the median nerve and the transverse carpal ligament are located and dissected. During the surgery, the median nerve is released by cutting the transverse carpal ligament and removing all the adhesions present along the nerve.

c. Finally, intraneural and perineural injections of PRP are performed. In addition, a fibrin membrane is placed between the nerve and the ligament, to later suture the incision.

5. Clinical results of PRP application for peripheral nerve injury

PRP products present a number of features that are quickening the application of this therapy in clinical practice, namely ease of use, reasonable biosafety and great versatility. Therefore, and although the PRP is still a recent technique, several clinical studies have emerging in the last decade (**Table 2**).

5.1 PRP infiltrations as conservative treatment

As in other pathologies, pain is one of the main problems of patients who suffer from peripheral nerve injuries. PRP showed to be a promising therapeutic tool for the relief or reduction of pain associated with neuropathies. Malahias et al. conducted a case series study where patients who suffered from carpal tunnel syndrome (CTS) were treated with one PRP US-guided injection around the median nerve [43]. At 3 months of follow-up, the pain was significantly alleviated in 11 out of 14 patients according to VAS score. A prospective controlled study carried out by Uzun et al. demonstrated the effectiveness of PRP in reducing the pain associated with CTS after one perineural injection of 2 mL of PRP [44]. These kinds of interventions were conducted not only over the median nerve but also over the ulnar nerve. Patients with peripheral neuropathy associated to leprosy received a perineural injection of 1 mL of PRP in the posterior tibial nerves and in the ulnar nerve. The results of this randomized control clinical trial showed a pain decrease 2 weeks after treatment [45].

These results are also accompanied by a functional and clinical improvement, which has a positive impact on the quality of life of patients. Some of the patients mentioned above showed functional recovery together with reduction in pain [42, 43]. More clinical studies also showed improvement in clinical and functional symptomatology when applying PRP in different peripheral nerve lesions. Recently, a randomized clinical study demonstrated better functional outcomes in patients with mild to moderate CTS [46]. Patients who received one US-guided infiltration of PRP into the carpal tunnel achieved a better response that patients treated with

Reference	Condition	Target	Intervention	Improvement
Infiltrations				
[43]	CTS	MN	US-guided perineural injection (1 × 1–2 mL)	Pain and function
[44]	CTS	MN	Perineural injection (1 × 2 mL)	Pain and function
[45]	Leprosy peripheral neuropathy	PTN and UN	Perineural injection (1 × 1 mL)	Pain
[46]	CTS	MN	US-guided perineural injection (1 × 1–2 mL)	Function
[47]	Perinatal cerebral palsy	Systemic	Intravenous injection (1 × 25 mL)	Function
[48]	CTS	MN	Injection at the distal carpal crease (1 × 1 mL)	Pain, function and EMG
[49]	CTS	MN	US-guided perineural injection (1 × 3 mL)	Pain, function and EMG
[50]	CPN palsy	CPN	US-guided intraneural/perineural infiltrations (13 × 3–8 mL)	Pain, function and EMG
[51]	CTS	MN	US-guided perineural injection (2 × 5 mL)	Pain, function and EMG
[52]	Section of RN	RN	US-guided intraneural injections (5 × 4 mL)	Function and EMG
Surgery				
[53]	Nerve gaps in extremities	Nerves of the extremities	Nerve gap bridged with a collagen tube with PRP fibrin	Function
[54]	Persistent pudendal neuralgia	PN	Injection after a transgluteal decompression	Function
[55]	Benign parotid gland tumor with facial muscles and nerve deficit	FN	PRP gel was applied around nerve endings during superficial parotidectomy	Function

CPN, common peroneal nerve; CTS, carpal tunnel syndrome; EMG, electromyography; FN, facial nerve; MN, median nerve; PRP, platelet-rich plasma; PTN, posterior tibial nerve; RN, radial nerve; UN, ulnar nerve; US, ultrasound.

Table 2.
Clinical research of PRP application for peripheral nerve injury.

saline 12 weeks after treatment. However, in this study, no differences in pain scores were found. A case report that described a 6-year-old boy with perinatal cerebral palsy should be noted [49]. After receiving an intravenous injection of 25 mL of PRP, an improvement in the cognitive sphere and language during the follow-up at 3 and 6 months was observed. Levels of GF maintained stable in plasma 3–5 times higher than average for his age group.

It must be taken into consideration that some variables may have a certain subjective component or be influenced by other factors than the treatment administered. Thus, it is advisable to analyze more objective variables such as EMG. A randomized controlled study showed improvement in EMG parameters, such as sensory nerve action potential (SNAP) in CTS patients [48]. However, there were no differences between control group (splint) and PRP treatment. This could be because the infiltration performed in this study was conducted without US guidance or directly into the median nerve but in adjacent areas, hampering the biological effects of PRP on the nervous tissue. Wu et al. carried out other randomized controlled study of CTS patients achieving an enhancement in sensory nerve conduction velocity (SNCV) and distal motor latency (DML) [49]. Although these EMG values were not significantly better than control group, there were significant differences in terms of pain and other clinical symptoms. The authors observed this improvement 6 months after one US-guided injection of 3 mL of PRP in the median nerve. In a case report described by Sánchez et al., a patient with peroneal nerve palsy underwent serial US-guided intraneural and perineural injections for 33 months [50]. The patient not only achieved improvement related to pain and function but also showed EMG sings of reinnervation for the peroneus longus and tibialis anterior. Specifically, an increase in compound muscle action (CMAP) was reported. In another case report, a 56-year-old woman who suffered from severity of symptoms of CTS received a treatment consisted of two US-guided perineural injections of 5 mL of PRP [51]. During follow-up at 3 and 6 months after the treatment, she revealed significant improvements in the distal motor and sensory latencies as well as the sensory nerve action potential and CMAP amplitudes of the median nerves. Finally, García de Cortazar et al. reported a case that described a patient with a section of the radial nerve [52]. Four months after the trauma and consequent surgery without positive response, serial intraneural infiltrations of PRP were conducted with US guidance. Eleven months after the first injection, EMG showed a complete reinnervation of the musculature of the radial nerve dependent.

5.2 PRP as adjuvant in surgery

In addition to the application of PRP in liquid form for neural infiltrations, its versatility allows it to formulate in different ways such as gel, scaffold or fibrin membrane to apply also in surgical interventions. (**Figure 1**). Kuffler et al. took advantage of these properties for patients with nerve gaps in their extremities [53]. In the surgical technique they conducted, collagen tubes filled with PRP formulated as fibrin membrane were used to bridge the nerve gaps. Patients of this case series reached sensory and motor recovery across nerve gap, reduction of pain and functional recovery. Hibner et al. observed in a retrospective analysis the efficacy of injecting PRP around the pudendal nerve after a transgluteal decompression to enclose the nerve in NeuroWrapNerve Protector [54]. The pain of these patients who suffered from persistent pudendal neuralgia after neurolysis and transposition was significantly alleviated. This success was also achieved in patients with facial muscle and nerve deficit associated with benign parotid gland tumor [55]. In this randomized control study, Scala et al. observed significant improvements in several clinical parameters in the group of patients where PRP gel was applied during superficial parotidectomy.

6. Conclusion

6.1 Final considerations

Neuropathies are very challenging pathologies whose treatment options include conservative procedures as well as surgical interventions. In both cases, PRP is a promising and safe therapeutic tool that can be used as liquid formulation for

US-guided infiltrations or as fibrin scaffold for surgery. Its potential has been proved in diverse in vitro and in vivo studies, and there are constantly more treatments based on this therapy in humans also. The use of this technique allows physicians to take advantage of the biological processes required to achieve an optimal nerve repair and satisfactory clinical results.

6.2 Future directions

Although the PRP application for nerve pathologies is showing encouraging results and no negative side effects, apart from some painful episodes during injections, its use in these pathologies still has to be cautious. Although in some treatments normally the employed product has its importance, the way to use this product is also relevant to achieve a successful response. Elements such as a correct indication, an appropriate PRP elaboration and a suitable administration and application procedures are essential for the success of these treatments. Further studies and cases are needed to increase the knowledge not only of PRP for neuropathies but also of nerve biology, and thus improve protocols as well as clinical outcomes.

Author details

Mikel Sánchez[1,2], Ane Garate[1], Ane Miren Bilbao[2], Jaime Oraa[2], Fernando Yangüela[2], Pello Sánchez[1], Jorge Guadilla[2], Beatriz Aizpurua[2], Juan Azofra[2], Nicolás Fiz[2] and Diego Delgado[1*]

1 Advanced Biological Therapy Unit, Hospital Vithas San José, Vitoria-Gasteiz, Spain

2 Arthroscopic Surgery Unit, Hospital Vithas San José, Vitoria-Gasteiz, Spain

*Address all correspondence to: diego.delgado@ucatrauma.com

References

[1] Sánchez M, Delgado D, Sánchez P, Fiz N, Azofra J, Orive G, et al. Platelet rich plasma and knee surgery. BioMed Research International. 2014;**2014**:890630. DOI: 10.1155/2014/890630

[2] Sánchez M, Anitua E, Delgado D, Sanchez P, Prado R, Orive G, et al. Platelet-rich plasma, a source of autologous growth factors and biomimetic scaffold for peripheral nerve regeneration. Expert Opinion on Biological Therapy. 2017;**17**(2):197-212. DOI: 10.1080/14712598.201

[3] Willits K, Kaniki N, Bryant D. The use of platelet-rich plasma in orthopedic injuries. Sports Medicine and Arthroscopy Review. 2013;**21**(4):225-230. DOI: 10.1097/JSA.0000000000000001

[4] Alves R, Grimalt R. A review of platelet-rich plasma: History, biology, mechanism of action, and classification. Skin Appendage Disorders. 2018;**4**(1):18-24. DOI: 10.1159/000477353

[5] Lopez E, Bermejo N, Berna-Erro A, Alonso N, Salido GM, Redondo PC, et al. A relationship between calcium mobilization and platelet α- and δ-granule secretion. A role for TRPC6 in thrombin-evoked δ-granule exocytosis. Archives of Biochemistry and Biophysics. 2015;**585**:75-81. DOI: 10.1016/j.abb.2015.09.012

[6] Scully D, Naseem KM, Matsakas A. Platelet biology in regenerative medicine of skeletal muscle. Acta Physiologica (Oxford, England). 2018:e13071. DOI: 10.1111/apha.13071

[7] Garate A, Sánchez P, Delgado D, Bilbao AM, Muiños-López E, Granero-Moltó F, et al. Autologous bioscaffolds based on different concentrations of platelet rich plasma and synovial fluid as a vehicle for mesenchymal stem cells. Journal of Biomedical Materials Research. Part A. 2018;**106**(2):377-385. DOI: 10.1002/jbm.a.36247

[8] Dohle E, El Bagdadi K, Sader R, Choukroun J, James Kirkpatrick C, Ghanaati S. Platelet-rich fibrin-based matrices to improve angiogenesis in an in vitro co-culture model for bone tissue engineering. Journal of Tissue Engineering and Regenerative Medicine. 2018;**12**(3):598-610. DOI: 10.1002/term.2475

[9] Sánchez M, Garate A, Delgado D, Padilla S. Platelet-rich plasma, an adjuvant biological therapy to assist peripheral nerve repair. Neural Regeneration Research. 2017;**12**(1):47-52. DOI: 10.4103/1673-5374.198973

[10] Koda M, Someya Y, Nishio Y, Kadota R, Mannoji C, Miyashita T, et al. Brain-derived neurotrophic factor suppresses anoikis-induced death of Schwann cells. Neuroscience Letters. 2008;**444**(2):143-147. DOI: 10.1016/j.neulet.2008.07.055

[11] Wang Z, Deng Q, Zhang X, Zhang J. Treatment of injured neurons with bone marrow stem cells cotransfected by hTERT and Ad-BDNF in vitro. Journal of Molecular Neuroscience. 2009;**38**(3):265-272. DOI: 10.1007/s12031-009-9208-5

[12] Zurita M, Otero L, Aguayo C, Bonilla C, Ferreira E, Parajón A, et al. Cell therapy for spinal cord repair: Optimization of biologic scaffolds for survival and neural differentiation of human bone marrow stromal cells. Cytotherapy. 2010;**12**(4):522-537. DOI: 10.3109/14653241003615164

[13] Apel PJ, Ma J, Callahan M, Northam CN, Alton TB, Sonntag WE, et al. Effect of locally delivered IGF-1 on nerve regeneration during aging: An experimental study in rats. Muscle

& Nerve. 2010;**41**(3):335-341. DOI: 10.1002/mus.21485

[14] Erlandsson A, Enarsson M, Forsberg-Nilsson K. Immature neurons from CNS stem cells proliferate in response to platelet-derived growth factor. The Journal of Neuroscience. 2001;**21**(10):3483-3491

[15] Luo H, Zhang Y, Zhang Z, Jin Y. The protection of MSCs from apoptosis in nerve regeneration by TGFβ1 through reducing inflammation and promoting VEGF-dependent angiogenesis. Biomaterials. 2012;**33**(17):4277-4287. DOI: 10.1016/j.biomaterials.2012.02.042

[16] Anitua E, Pascual C, Pérez-Gonzalez R, Orive G, Carro E. Intranasal PRGF-Endoret enhances neuronal survival and attenuates NF-κB-dependent inflammation process in a mouse model of Parkinson's disease. Journal of Controlled Release. 2015;**203**:170-180. DOI: 10.1016/j.jconrel.2015.02.030

[17] Li S, Gu X, Yi S. The regulatory effects of transforming growth factor-β on nerve regeneration. Cell Transplantation. 2017;**26**(3):381-394. DOI: 10.3727/096368916X693824

[18] Rosenstein JM, Krum JM. New roles for VEGF in nervous tissue—Beyond blood vessels. Experimental Neurology. 2004;**187**(2):246-253

[19] Yu CQ, Zhang M, Matis KI, Kim C, Rosenblatt MI. Vascular endothelial growth factor mediates corneal nerve repair. Investigative Ophthalmology & Visual Science. 2008;**49**(9):3870-3878. DOI: 10.1167/iovs.07-1418

[20] Borselli C, Storrie H, Benesch-Lee F, Shvartsman D, Cezar C, Lichtman JW, et al. Functional muscle regeneration with combined delivery of angiogenesis and myogenesis factors. Proceedings of the National Academy of Sciences of the United States of America. 2010;**107**(8):3287-3292. DOI: 10.1073/pnas.0903875106

[21] Kim JY, Jeon WJ, Kim DH, Rhyu IJ, Kim YH, Youn I, et al. An inside-out vein graft filled with platelet-rich plasma for repair of a short sciatic nerve defect in rats. Neural Regeneration Research. 2014;**9**(14):1351-1357. DOI: 10.4103/1673-5374.137587

[22] Ceccarelli J, Putnam AJ. Sculpting the blank slate: How fibrin's support of vascularization can inspire biomaterial design. Acta Biomaterialia. 2014;**10**(4):1515-1523. DOI: 10.1016/j.actbio.2013.07.043

[23] Zheng C, Zhu Q, Liu X, Huang X, He C, Jiang L, et al. Effect of platelet-rich plasma (PRP) concentration on proliferation, neurotrophic function and migration of Schwann cells in vitro. Journal of Tissue Engineering and Regenerative Medicine. 2016;**10**(5):428-436. DOI: 10.1002/term.1756

[24] Takeuchi M, Kamei N, Shinomiya R, Sunagawa T, Suzuki O, Kamoda H, et al. Human platelet-rich plasma promotes axon growth in brain-spinal cord coculture. Neuroreport. 2012;**23**(12):712-716. DOI: 10.1097/WNR.0b013e3283567196

[25] Ye F, Li H, Qiao G, Chen F, Tao H, Ji A, et al. Platelet-rich plasma gel in combination with Schwann cells for repair of sciatic nerve injury. Neural Regeneration Research. 2012;**7**(29):2286-2292. DOI: 10.3969/j.issn.1673-5374.2012.29.007

[26] Yu W, Wang J, Yin J. Platelet-rich plasma: A promising product for treatment of peripheral nerve regeneration after nerve injury. The International Journal of Neuroscience. 2011;**121**(4):176-180. DOI: 10.3109/00207454.2010.544432

[27] Cho HH, Jang S, Lee SC, Jeong HS, Park JS, Han JY, et al. Effect of

neural-induced mesenchymal stem cells and platelet-rich plasma on facial nerve regeneration in an acute nerve injury model. The Laryngoscope. 2010;**120**(5):907-913. DOI: 10.1002/lary.20860

[28] Lichtenfels M, Colomé L, Sebben AD, Braga-Silva J. Effect of platelet rich plasma and platelet rich fibrin on sciatic nerve regeneration in a rat model. Microsurgery. 2013;**33**(5):383-390. DOI: 10.1002/micr.22105

[29] Ma CH, Omura T, Cobos EJ, Latrémolière A, Ghasemlou N, Brenner GJ, et al. Accelerating axonal growth promotes motor recovery after peripheral nerve injury in mice. The Journal of Clinical Investigation. 2011;**121**(11):4332-4347. DOI: 10.1172/JCI58675

[30] Sánchez M, Anitua E, Delgado D, Prado R, Sánchez P, Fiz N, et al. Ultrasound-guided plasma rich in growth factors injections and scaffolds hasten motor nerve functional recovery in an ovine model of nerve crush injury. Journal of Tissue Engineering and Regenerative Medicine. 2017;**11**(5):1619-1629. DOI: 10.1002/term.2079

[31] Sariguney Y, Yavuzer R, Elmas C, Yenicesu I, Bolay H, Atabay K. Effect of platelet-rich plasma on peripheral nerve regeneration. Journal of Reconstructive Microsurgery. 2008;**24**(3):159-167. DOI: 10.1055/s-2008-1076752

[32] Anitua E, Pelacho B, Prado R, Aguirre JJ, Sánchez M, Padilla S, et al. Infiltration of plasma rich in growth factors enhances in vivo angiogenesis and improves reperfusion and tissue remodeling after severe hind limb ischemia. Journal of Controlled Release. 2015;**202**:31-39. DOI: 10.1016/j.jconrel.2015.01.029

[33] Schaakxs D, Kalbermatten DF, Raffoul W, Wiberg M, Kingham PJ. Regenerative cell injection in denervated muscle reduces atrophy and enhances recovery following nerve repair. Muscle & Nerve. 2013;**47**(5):691-701. DOI: 10.1002/mus.23662

[34] Shavlakadze T, White JD, Davies M, Hoh JF, Grounds MD. Insulin-like growth factor I slows the rate of denervation induced skeletal muscle atrophy. Neuromuscular Disorders. 2005;**15**(2):139-146. DOI: 10.1016/j.nmd.2004.10.013

[35] Giusti I, D'Ascenzo S, Mancò A, Di Stefano G, Di Francesco M, Rughetti A, et al. Platelet concentration in platelet-rich plasma affects tenocyte behavior in vitro. BioMed Research International. 2014;**2014**:630870. DOI: 10.1155/2014/630870

[36] Xu Z, Yin W, Zhang Y, Qi X, Chen Y, Xie X, et al. Comparative evaluation of leukocyte- and platelet-rich plasma and pure platelet-rich plasma for cartilage regeneration. Scientific Reports. 2017;**7**:43301. DOI: 10.1038/srep43301

[37] Sen O, Sayilgan NC, Tutuncu AC, Bakan M, Koksal GM, Oz H. Evaluation of sciatic nerve damage following intraneural injection of bupivacaine, levobupivacaine and lidocaine in rats. Brazilian Journal of Anesthesiology. 2016;**66**(3):272-275. DOI: 10.1016/j.bjane.2014.09.012

[38] Choquet O, Morau D, Biboulet P, Capdevila X. Where should the tip of the needle be located in ultrasound-guided peripheral nerve blocks? Current Opinion in Anaesthesiology. 2012;**25**(5):596-602. DOI: 10.1097/ACO.0b013e328356bb40

[39] Damjanovska M, Cvetko E, Hadzic A, Seliskar A, Plavec T, Mis K, et al. Neurotoxicity of perineural vs intraneural-extrafascicular injection of liposomal bupivacaine in the porcine model of sciatic nerve block. Anaesthesia. 2015;**70**(12):1418-1426. DOI: 10.1111/anae.13189

[40] Hasanbegovic I, Kulenovic A, Hasanovic S. Effects of intraneural and perineural injection and concentration of Ropivacaine on nerve injury during peripheral nerve block in Wistar rats. Journal of Health Sciences. 2013;**3**(3):243-249. DOI: 10.17532/jhsci.2013.115

[41] Brierley JB, Field EJ. The fate of an intraneural injection as demonstrated by the use of radio-active phosphorus. Journal of Neurology, Neurosurgery, and Psychiatry. 1949;**12**(2):86-99

[42] Cass SP. Ultrasound-guided nerve hydrodissection: What is it? A review of the literature. Current Sports Medicine Reports. 2016;**15**(1):20-22. DOI: 10.1249/JSR.0000000000000226

[43] Malahias MA, Johnson EO, Babis GC, Nikolaou VS. Single injection of platelet-rich plasma as a novel treatment of carpal tunnel syndrome. Neural Regeneration Research. 2015;**10**(11):1856-1859. DOI: 10.4103/1673-5374.165322

[44] Uzun H, Bitik O, Uzun Ö, Ersoy US, Aktaş E. Platelet-rich plasma versus corticosteroid injections for carpal tunnel syndrome. Journal of Plastic Surgery and Hand Surgery. 2017;**51**(5):301-305. DOI: 10.1080/2000656X.2016.1260025

[45] Anjayani S, Wirohadidjojo YW, Adam AM, Suwandi D, Seweng A, Amiruddin MD. Sensory improvement of leprosy peripheral neuropathy in patients treated with perineural injection of platelet-rich plasma. International Journal of Dermatology. 2014;**53**(1):109-113. DOI: 10.1111/ijd.12162

[46] Malahias MA, Nikolaou VS, Johnson EO, Kaseta MK, Kazas ST, Babis GC. Platelet-rich plasma ultrasound-guided injection in the treatment of carpal tunnel syndrome: A placebo-controlled clinical study. Journal of Tissue Engineering and Regenerative Medicine. 2018;**12**(3):e1480-e1488. DOI: 10.1002/term.2566

[47] Alcaraz J, Oliver A, Sánchez JM. Platelet-rich plasma in a patient with cerebral palsy. American Journal of Case Reports. 2015;**16**:469-472. DOI: 10.12659/AJCR.893805

[48] Raeissadat SA, Karimzadeh A, Hashemi M, Bagherzadeh L. Safety and efficacy of platelet-rich plasma in treatment of carpal tunnel syndrome; a randomized controlled trial. BMC Musculoskeletal Disorders. 2018;**19**(1):49. DOI: 10.1186/s12891-018-1963-4

[49] Wu YT, Ho TY, Chou YC, Ke MJ, Li TY, Huang GS, et al. Six-month efficacy of platelet-rich plasma for carpal tunnel syndrome: A prospective randomized, single-blind controlled trial. Scientific Reports. 2017;**7**(1):94. DOI: 10.1038/s41598-017-00224-6

[50] Sánchez M, Yoshioka T, Ortega M, Delgado D, Anitua E. Ultrasound-guided platelet-rich plasma injections for the treatment of common peroneal nerve palsy associated with multiple ligament injuries of the knee. Knee Surgery, Sports Traumatology, Arthroscopy. 2014;**22**(5):1084-1089. DOI: 10.1007/s00167-013-2479-y

[51] Kuo YC, Lee CC, Hsieh LF. Ultrasound-guided perineural injection with platelet-rich plasma improved the neurophysiological parameters of carpal tunnel syndrome: A case report. Journal of Clinical Neuroscience. 2017;**44**:234-236. DOI: 10.1016/j.jocn.2017.06.053

[52] García de Cortázar U, Padilla S, Lobato E, Delgado D, Sánchez M. Intraneural platelet-rich plasma injections for the treatment of radial nerve section: A case report. Journal of Clinical Medicine. 2018;**7**(2):pii:E13. DOI: 10.3390/jcm7020013

[53] Kuffler DP. An assessment of current techniques for inducing axon regeneration and neurological recovery following peripheral nerve trauma. Progress in Neurobiology. 2014;**116**:1-12. DOI: 10.1016/j.pneurobio.2013.12.004

[54] Hibner M, Castellanos ME, Drachman D, Balducci J. Repeat operation for treatment of persistent pudendal nerve entrapment after pudendal neurolysis. Journal of Minimally Invasive Gynecology. 2012;**19**(3):325-330. DOI: 10.1016/j.jmig.2011.12.022

[55] Scala M, Mereu P, Spagnolo F, Massa M, Barla A, Mosci S, et al. The use of platelet-rich plasma gel in patients with mixed tumour undergoing superficial parotidectomy: A randomized study. In Vivo. 2014;**28**(1):121-124